The Inner Pulse

The Inner Pulse

*Unlocking the Secret Code
of Sickness and Health*

MARC SIEGEL, M.D.

WILEY

John Wiley & Sons, Inc.

Published by John Wiley & Sons, Inc., Hoboken, New Jersey
Published simultaneously in Canada

For general information about our other products and services, please contact our Customer Care Department within the United States at (800) 762–2974, outside the United States at (317) 572–3993 or fax (317) 572–4002.

Wiley also publishes its books in a variety of electronic formats. Some content that appears in print may not be available in electronic books. For more information about Wiley products, visit our web site at www.wiley.com.

Library of Congress Cataloging-in-Publication Data:

Siegel, Marc (Marc K.)
    The inner pulse : unlocking the secret code of sickness and health / Marc Siegel.
       p. ; cm.
    Includes bibliographical references and index.
    ISBN 978-0-470-26039-5 (cloth : alk. paper); ISBN 978-1-118-02806-3 (ebk);
    ISBN 978-1-118-02807-0 (ebk); ISBN 978-1-118-02808-7 (ebk)
       1. Mental healing. 2. Health–Psychological aspects. 3. Mind and body. I. Title.
    [DNLM: 1. Mental Healing. 2. Attitude to Health. 3. Mind-Body Relations,
    Metaphysical. 4. Patients–psychology. 5. Volition. WB 880]
    RZ400.S622 2011
    615.8'51–dc22

                                                                            2010054048

Printed in the United States of America

10 9 8 7 6 5 4 3 2 1

To my mother and father, Annette and Bernard,
who conceived my inner pulse

Faith is the sense of life, that sense by virtue of which man does not destroy himself but continues to live on. It is the force whereby we live.

—*Leo Tolstoy*

Contents

Preface xi

Acknowledgments xvii

Introduction 1

PART ONE: Knowing Your Inner Pulse

1 Surgeons of the Mind 9

2 The Pulse of Recovery 15

3 One Patient, Many Pulses 29

4 Inner Pulse Rising 43

5 Radar to Die 59

PART TWO: The Healing Pulse

6 Dancing in the Dark 73

7 Infection of Body, Infection of Spirit 87

8 Never Say Die 95

9 Radar to Live 111

10   The Black Swan   121

11   The Truth about Psychic Healing   133

PART THREE: The Pulse of Power

12   The Strongest Inner Pulse   145

13   Who Dies? Who Lives?   155

14   Considering the Alternative   167

15   Miracles and the Inner Pulse   173

Afterword: All in Good Time   187

Bibliography   197
Recommended Reading   221
Index   223

Preface

I have always wanted to understand the emotional component of illness and recovery. Long before I became a physician, I came to the realization that there is an essential life force inside all of us that grows stronger with good health and weaker with disease. I couldn't really comprehend or define this force, but I knew that it was fundamental and that it could disappear in an instant, causing death. I have been fascinated by this phenomenon since I was a child, and I pursued a greater awareness of it as I grew into adulthood.

My Jewish great-grandparents were murdered in a pogrom in Poland at the turn of the twentieth century. This horrific event forever changed my family in ways that related to body, mind, and spirit. I wanted to understand what happened and how I could use that understanding to help others.

This led me to enter the practice of medicine from an unusual angle, one closer to humanism than to pure science. In the course of my medical training, I began to recognize a previously undescribed force as a kind of radar for wellness, a spiritual and physical element that exists deep within us—invisible and immeasurable, yet central to all of our lives. I came to call this force the inner pulse.

As a doctor, I began to consider the pulse. Sometimes I thought I could tame it or change it. I came to realize that controlling this nameless unseen power is very difficult. It shapes us much more than we can shape it. Apprehending the power of the inner pulse is the most that many of us can do.

Sensing the inner pulse can help a patient or a doctor predict, much more than alter, the future. The inner pulse is a harbinger of future events, illness, and death, as well as recovery and cure. Masters and healers ply their various physical disciplines and treatments, as well as mental concentration techniques, to effect a subtle change. In extraordinary cases, a major change occurs.

A person can learn to know his or her inner pulse much better than any physician can, although a good physician can learn to be attentive through a career of careful listening. A good doctor is always trying to sense this pulse.

A chance experience that occurred before I entered medical school prepared me to become sensitive and receptive to the uncanny world of strange and unexpected cures.

In 1976, at the age of twenty, I rode my bicycle across the United States and Canada with my best friend, Ron. We rode more than a hundred miles a day east across the Canadian Rockies and onto the plains of Alberta, pushing ourselves to our physical limits. We soon found that succeeding at this pace required an intense focus.

As we pedaled in an accelerated rhythm for hour after hour, our perceptions became heightened and we entered a trance-like state. We rarely spoke, and the world around us seemed increasingly strange and foreign. Almost every morning we awoke in our campsites to a cloudy or drizzly sky with a swarm of black flies settling over us. Almost every afternoon, while riding our bicycles, we watched the blanket of black clouds that covered the sky from horizon to horizon and hoped for even a slant of sunshine. We wore drab plastic ponchos that did not keep us dry. The top of my tan poncho acted as a funnel, and the rainwater collected on the bridge of my nose and dripped onto my chin and down my neck.

Alberta was desolate. Route 1 was a major cross-Canadian route, yet we rode for several hours at around fifteen miles an hour without seeing another human being. We held a running conversation to stay alert. We lived the primitive realities of the land and the sky and the search for food and a place to sleep every night.

One day in late July, riding along Route 1, Ron and I were caught up in a discussion about the purpose of our lives. It was approaching twilight, and the shadows of bicycle and rider were lengthening on the road when all of a sudden the long accelerating shadow of a station wagon appeared on the horizon behind us. It was the first car we had seen in more than five hours. As we looked over our left shoulders and saw the bright metal car, Ron and I felt instinctively that we were in trouble—it was something we could intuit from the way the vehicle was speeding, yet drifting in its lane. I began to move to the side of the road and onto the shoulder. Ron, having the same feeling, did the same.

Less than a hundred yards from us, the driver lost control. The skids along the dry road made a sharp, screeching sound. I was startled—my midbrain sent a message to my nerves and muscles to initiate a fight or flight response. My amygdala, the emotional center of the primitive deep brain, authorized a surge of adrenaline and noradrenaline, and my jazzed-up reflexes instantly caused me to jump from the road and as far down into the small ravine by the side as I could go. Pressed against the embankment there, joined by Ron, our hearts racing from the hormones, we waited, staring straight ahead as the out-of-control car skidded and careened along. Finally, the images of our shadows on the road converged. The car shadow missed the shadows of our heads and bodies and bicycles by inches. Once past, the car skidded wildly a few more times until the driver slowed, regained control, and continued on. He didn't stop.

Ron and I looked at each other, shaken yet relieved that we had saved ourselves with a reflexive leap from the road. Probability would never have anticipated either the problem— that the car would lose control—or the only possible solution. Our inner pulses saved our lives.

The nearly fatal accident on that Alberta road became my first major step in the direction of becoming a healing physician. We had anticipated an unlikely event. We had been provoked to action by a deep intuition that defied science. The mental process could not have been learned in any classroom.

As the stories in this book show, the real understanding of how a treatment works often come's from a deep intuition connected to the inner pulse. During my two decades as a physician, I have learned to work with the interior lives of my patients. A crucial aspect of the inner pulse is that it can simultaneously reveal or anticipate an awful illness or event, while at the same time point to and help forge the path to recovery. It is the sign of something going wrong, yet it also fuels the courage and perseverance needed for a cure. An astute patient can feel both the surge of life and the precipice of death simultaneously.

As I have grown into a healer, not merely a physician, I have begun to look for clues beyond my preconceptions and the medical facts of a case to determine the cause of a patient's suffering.

I have learned to be empathetic with a sick person and look for his or her moral directive—and to unlock my own emotions.

I speak from the personal experience of having overcome a negative force in my own mind. I was a patient myself, and I will describe my struggle in the first chapter of this book.

I hope I have become the kind of doctor who listens to and heeds his patients' inner pulses. This book presents the tortuous path that got me there. Along the way, I encountered many nondoctors who were far ahead of me in understanding the inner pulse. Mystical rabbis, priests, psychics, and many others of varying perspectives and fields of expertise have learned to apprehend and sometimes even influence the pulse. Throughout this book, I provide examples of patients who benefited directly from these healers. I have changed the names of my patients and other doctors who treated them as well as the names of nurses and aides to protect their privacy. I use the real names of experts I interviewed or whose work I refer to.

Always remember: if you tap into your inner pulse, it will lead the way forward.

Acknowledgments

In uncovering the inner pulse, I have found that it manifests itself in completely different ways in different people. Learning to recognize and work with your own inner pulse is an essential way to cope and to function effectively as part of life's many teams.

The same is true of constructing a successful book. The essential ingredients of this or any book vary from family to friend to editor to agent, each with a different, crucial role. The blend in this case has led to the creation of an extremely original, yet well-integrated, fabric. Tom Miller, Executive Editor of General Interest books at John Wiley & Sons, is a highly creative, work-through-the-night type of editor with the kind of commitment and passion for his books that is matched only by those of his authors. Miller ran my manuscript through his selective editorial *mill* repeatedly, testing the product for soundness, cohesiveness, structural integrity, and above all, quality. He took a vital and personal interest in the health and recovery issues addressed in this book, and his devotion helped the book enormously. A writer is very lucky when he can say that his editor is this indispensable to a book's success.

Tom's senior editorial assistant, Jorge Amaral, is a perfect complement to Tom, organized and attentive to details, responsive to author frustrations, and a good sounding board for ideas.

Wiley's production was handled by Senior Production Editor John Simko, who does a fantastic job of pruning, cleaning, and weeding a manuscript—detail-oriented in the best sense.

Mike Onorato, head of publicity for General Interest books at Wiley and a longtime friend, is an unending resource of ideas in terms of book promotion and diplomacy, and I am grateful for his consistent support and encouragement over the years.

Kitt Allan, my publisher, has an inner pulse of the highest order, a spiritual blend of calm kindness combined with the brawn of business know-how and literary creativity. She has been a great backstop for this book and, along with Tom, has added greatly to its vision and passion.

Gail Ross and Howard Yoon, my agents, have stuck by me throughout the project and have stayed calm and practical, keeping their eyes on the goal. As my media platform has grown via Fox News, Sirius/XM, and the *Los Angeles Times*, they have recognized the growing opportunity to bring this book to a large audience who will appreciate a fresh approach to their health.

The Johnsons are my second family, a constant source of support and succor. Roger Ailes, my boss at Fox News, not only has a big inner pulse, he also has a great heart. I also want to thank my friend Bill Shine, head of programming at Fox News, for all his kindness and support. Dean Robert Grossman, my boss at NYU Langone Medical Center, is also a man of great instinct and vision.

The Inner Pulse is a real life story of patients and doctors embarked on a course of discovery, enlightenment, and struggle. I want to thank my patients (including my father and father-in-law) for participating. I have changed the names of my patients and the names of the other doctors, nurses, and aids who helped me treat them. (I have kept the real names of the physicians I interviewed or cited as experts). I have camouflaged details in order to preserve privacy. But without my patients and their personal stories, I would not have a book, and I am grateful to them.

Finally, I want to thank my family. My wife, Luda, is not only a great wife and mother who has great forbearance when it comes to her husband, but as this book also illustrates, she is a brilliant doctor. I know no better diagnostician, and when patients admit to me that they prefer her kind manner to my own, I accept it as a compliment.

The Inner Pulse

Introduction

What is the inner pulse?

The inner pulse indicates whether the life force is fading or strengthening. It is the strongest power in the body, and it helps determine both living and dying. Although it cannot be measured, it can be sensed. It is the fulcrum of a person's life force, the place where the physical and the spiritual combine. It is the link between your body's life force and your soul, tangible proof of your connection to a larger reality and of that reality's strong presence in your body.

The inner pulse surges with your life force; it fades and stops with your death. When you are dead, the inner pulse is gone, but your soul persists.

Is there a benefit to being aware of your inner pulse? There is indeed. Knowing your inner pulse can mean knowing the direction your health is heading. If your pulse creates a foreboding sense that you are in jeopardy, there may still be time for you to undergo treatments and make changes in your life that can potentially save you. If "objective" medical tests predict a likely bad outcome, your inner pulse may still inform you that you have some chance to survive. Conversely, even if medical science reassures you that nothing is wrong, your inner pulse may alert you that something terrible is about to happen. The inner pulse is more than just instinct and intuition.

This book includes many stories of people I have treated and known whose destinies have been affected by an awareness of their inner pulse. My twenty-three-year-old patient Ann, for example, knew that something was horribly wrong, that her back pain was more than simply back pain. Before she became my patient, she had been referred to specialists who ranged from orthopedists to neurologists, and she was given muscle relaxants and ibuprofen, but she knew that something still wasn't right. Finally, a CT scan confirmed her worst suspicions: she had ovarian cancer, which was discovered just in time for surgery to be effective and bring about a complete cure.

Clearly, being aware of the inner pulse can change your life dramatically in a positive way. You will likely experience maximum benefit after years of careful listening to your body's signals or patterns. You will learn that whenever a disturbance occurs in the usual rhythm of your inner pulse, it may be a sign of impending illness, which you can then hopefully prepare for. Of course, knowing your pulse does not in any way undermine or replace the science-based treatments prescribed to help you, though the pulse can help you sense or even predict your response.

As a doctor, when I sense an inner pulse grow faint, I am alerted to the narrow window of time that I may still have to save the patient. Although medical schools don't study the inner pulse and residencies don't train doctors to respond to it, the art of sensing the inner pulse may be my most powerful medical tool by far.

A gifted physician, spiritual healer, or psychic can sometimes shape the pulse by focusing a concentrated healing force on a patient. Unfortunately, too many doctors lack the ability to either apprehend the inner pulse or influence it in any way. An astute patient can sense that such a doctor is out of touch with this vital force. A patient may feel as if he has a sense of his own pulse, but the average doctor, unless he or she is exceptionally intuitive or observant, rarely does.

My friend Lori, a thirty-year-old journalist, spent almost a year trying to figure out why she felt so weak, nauseous, and unfocused, until an astute physician in Boston, with his ear to her inner pulse, discovered an eight-pound adrenal tumor that other doctors had failed to find. She underwent a successful surgical cure.

I believe that only a career of unconventional and purposeful listening to many patients can enable a doctor to become a true spiritual healer with the ability to monitor the patient's inner pulse as part of a comprehensive practice of medicine. There are hints and clues to follow, paths to an untimely end or a timely cure that are not readily discernible by the inexperienced eye. These clues can only be detected by a sensitive doctor.

Medical school does not prepare its fledgling doctors to consider the uncanny world of unseen forces. Unlike traditional Asian systems of medicine, which focus on subtle energies such as prana or chi and their pathways through the body, traditional Western medical education emphasizes rote training and imprinting. The deep emotional and psychic components of illness are all too often ignored by text and teacher. It is not surprising that when we graduate, we doctors find that our medical tools are inadequate. Lacking awareness of the inner pulse, doctors are unprepared to handle the unexpected miraculous cure or the seemingly bizarre unpredicted death.

Unempirical, difficult-to-map experiences rarely appear in the scientific literature, but they often occur in people's lives. Kenneth Hammond, a noted psychologist, speaks of "a cognitive process that somehow produces an answer, solution, or idea without the use of a conscious, logically defensible step-by-step process." That answer, that solution, may be found in listening to the inner pulse. Deep intuition may provide access to the inner pulse. In her book *Educating Intuition*, Robin Hogarth wrote that intuition is a form of expertise and should be treated as such: "It is acquired through . . . experience. And it can be improved through instruction and practice."

Unfortunately, rather than using intuition to dig deeper and discover the inner pulse in their quest for health, patients who find no outlet for their emotions or intuition in the modern world of medical science may run away entirely from tested treatments and enter the often untested world of alternative medicine (whose remedies are sometimes valuable, other times not), never to return to traditional healing. It is because so many doctors do not learn from, or pay attention to, our patients' natural insights and instincts regarding their inner pulse that hucksters can swoop in and fill the void. These "healers" take the place of real doctors, in part because so many of our patients are disillusioned about the lack of emotional connection they experience with traditional practitioners.

Alternative medicine versus allopathic medicine—I will explore both sides of this important coin. I espouse a philosophy of health that is based on deep intuition combined with undeniable facts. I am not married to the mainstream viewpoint. I have traditional training, but I believe I have an expanded orientation.

Mainstream doctors do not become open overnight to the power of the mind and the role of emotions on health. Science provides treatments and mostly determines outcomes, but good health is more than the sum of these parts. We doctors don't generally leave the straight and narrow path of modern medicine unless we've had a variety of experiences that broaden our perspective.

In *Medical Miracles*, hematologist and believer Jacalyn Duffin reminds us of the connection between medicine and miracle cures and of how narrow-minded our medical training leads us to be. A miracle cure may be seen as the inner pulse dramatically manifesting in an unexpected healing. Duffin argues for openness to the spiritual world and concludes that sick people "may see doctors as instruments of healing, but they are equally comfortable, if not more inclined to, the opinion that real cures are effected by ourselves, by nature, or by deities with help from saints and long-lost predecessors. Getting better is directly connected to gestures of personal history, lifestyle, sacrifice, supplication, penance, and worship." Duffin's argument is impossible to prove. Though I disagree with directly mixing the scientific and spiritual worlds and using them as a guide to treatment, at the same time I don't think Duffin should be dismissed, either.

Having a sense of the subtle, unseen world began to help me as a physician as soon as I recognized that uncanny events may cluster around illness as markers of either death or recovery. The power of emotions may even have an impact on healing. When I realized this, I became more conscious of being kind and sensitive to my patients with regard to the quality and comprehensiveness of my treatments.

Healing requires that we discard rigid preconceived roles. These days, my insights and solutions come directly from my patients. I am not the person in charge. I am merely taking a patient's inner pulse and allowing it to help guide me. I cannot measure it, but I can learn to recognize it in its various guises. Over the years, I have learned to develop the flexibility to allow my patients to use their intuition to help predict the path to a cure.

Knowing about the inner pulse can be a great benefit to doctors and patients alike. In this book, I will go deep beneath the surface of the traditional doctor-patient interaction, and I will share with you what I find: stories and lessons of unexpected dilemmas, deaths, miracles, and cures.

PART ONE

Knowing Your Inner Pulse

It is not in the stars to hold our destiny but in ourselves.

—*William Shakespeare*

1

Surgeons of the Mind

A man should learn to detect and watch that gleam of light which flashes across his mind from within.

—Ralph Waldo Emerson

M ost of the time the inner pulse is first recognized after the fact, after an amazing event, a miracle, an unexpected recovery, or an unpredicted death has occurred. It is only then that a person looks in the rearview mirror at his or her erratic illness and realizes that scientific explanations may be insufficient. This experience can benefit a patient going forward by teaching him or her to recognize the inner pulse earlier in the healing process. Compiling these experiences among patients and learning from them can help a doctor become a true healer.

In 1997, I was newly married, and we had a newborn son, Joshua. My first novel had just been accepted for publication. I also moved into a new apartment for the first time in twelve years and simultaneously relocated my medical office. These sudden changes in my previously well-established routines helped throw me into a confused state. When there is a newborn in the house, the mother naturally shifts her affection, and not all new husbands can anticipate or handle this.

My son's middle-of-the-night cries combined with my growing unease, and I was soon awake for hours and unable to get back to sleep. I worried that this tiny being was too fragile to survive. I watched his miniscule chest rise and fall, and sometimes I was afraid to divert my glance for fear that when I looked at him again, he would be completely still, a SIDS baby.

This cycle of sleeplessness and increased worry triggered by the birth of my new son caused me to become depressed and anxious. In my later book *False Alarm*, I came to call this a cycle of worry. As I got worse, I obsessed on the growing strangeness in my life. I lost track of my inner pulse and was quickly on the defensive, just trying to finish the day without feeling more vulnerable than when the day started. Little felt real to me.

I was working on a revision of my novel and would fall asleep while working and awaken elsewhere in my apartment, not knowing how I got there. I was reacting to the stress of writing to a deadline, while living in a new apartment with a new child. Was I walking in my sleep, or was this some kind of trance? I worried that I could do some harm to my newborn if I picked him up while not fully awake. I consulted a sleep expert, who said that my sleeping problems were part of the anxiety I was experiencing. My inner pulse was fading, and I saw no easy path to recovery.

I grew more unhappy. I found that I didn't want to get out of bed in the morning. I saw a therapist, who suggested antidepressants. It is well known in psychiatry that worry and self-doubt can lead to more self-doubt, and I soon became concerned that my wife was no longer interested in me. In reality, she had physically withdrawn from me because her body still hadn't recovered from childbirth. I began to mention my concerns about my wife to my friends. At first this made me feel better, but then I worried that my friends might think less of me as a result. My deepest intuition alerted me that I was being irrational. I learned that anxiety isn't really a simple problem—it is mushrooming agony.

Psychotherapy wasn't helping. My therapist, Dr. Joseph Henson, a world-famous doctor, later admitted that he was so taken aback by my unexpected predicament that he responded to it with his own growing anxiety. His nervousness interfered with his ability to understand or help me.

The day I finally completed the manuscript for my novel, I tried to print it out for the publisher but couldn't find a working printer in my office. I became so upset that I sat at my desk for hours, unwilling to leave the office.

My wife began to consider leaving me. I was sleeping on the couch most nights, but the threat of divorce was a galvanizing moment that shocked me to change my behavior. From that point forward, I slowly learned to follow my inner pulse. One of the biggest shortcuts to health I had overlooked was my sense of humor, which is a deep remedy for all illness, especially psychiatric.

Dr. Henson had convinced himself that I would spend my life in stages of anxiety, self-doubt, and unhappiness. I never accepted Henson's assessment. Resisting the validity of his view turned out to be a key to the first stage of my recovery.

I switched to Dr. Arnold Knapp, a soft-spoken therapist from Columbia University with worn armchairs in his office and stacks of old unread medical journals on his couch. Dr. Knapp intuitively believed that my problems arose from adjusting to a new life and a massive mid-life crisis. He didn't feel that I required antidepressants.

Knapp's belief in me had a placebo effect. Knapp himself was the placebo. He drew an imaginary line and told me that on one side was disturbed thinking and that I was on the other side, in the world of worried neurosis. His analysis reassured me and helped me use my mental power to create a larger comfort zone. Once he had planted this seed, he encouraged it to grow. I replaced my self-doubts, one at a time, with a growing courage. Knapp prescribed self-control and self-esteem instead of pills. I believed in Knapp's intuitive truth, and I began to recover my health. My anxiety abated, my moods became more constant, and my mental wounds began to heal. There is a firm line in psychiatry between delusion—a locked vault of self-referring ideas that trap you and can agitate you—and the world of neurosis, where I was. Dr. Knapp helped me explore the world of the self-defeating neurotic. I could either continue to make myself miserable in that world, as so many others do, or I could be cured by therapy and relearn how to cope through fresh insights, guided by my inner pulse and by new teachers. Even on my most sleep-deprived days, I became less rigid and circumspect. I stopped fighting my wife for my son's affection and began to rebuild my relationship with her. I found that acting calm ultimately led to my feeling calm and that acting well ultimately led to my feeling well.

Healing is almost as painful as the illness, because scars, physical or psychological, are broken and replaced with healthy tissue. I relearned to project a businesslike aspect through my daily medical persona, even while I was still boiling up inside. Eventually, I became the professional I at first merely pretended to be. My emotions evened out. My healing current gradually gained traction.

While I was in the middle of my recovery, I became more religious. One Saturday morning, on the Jewish Sabbath, I passed a man outside my apartment who was saying a prayer in Hebrew for the birth of his son. I borrowed the prayer book and said a prayer for my own son. With my recovery, my wife softened, and I stayed with my small family.

Was my recovery a miracle? I have had no real anxiety for more than ten years. Few doctors would have either predicted this or been able to prescribe the many tiny progressive behavioral steps I took to strengthen myself. In retrospect, I would say that each of these steps was guided by my strengthening inner pulse and a faith in a higher power.

Was this a miracle in the religious sense? That is a hard question to answer. My recovery, though unconventional, certainly lacked the flash and fire that many would tend to associate with extraordinary religious miracles. Yet in the sense of a cure that defied scientific expectations and was driven by a connection to a greater spiritual reality, it was a miracle.

Viktor Frankl believed that a search for inner meaning helps mankind survive, even in the midst of the great suffering of the concentration camps he experienced and wrote about. Whether it is the power of the mind as triggered by a placebo or a connection to a divine being that triggers a miraculous improvement and a will to live, the effects should not be minimized.

As I recovered my balance and my place in the world, overcoming and escaping my deep midlife crisis, I felt as if I was being liberated from a prison of my own devising. As I regained my purpose and renewed my search for meaning, I read about the ancient Indian healing medical system called Ayurveda, which sees man as seeking to achieve a mental and physical balance between his structure, his function, and the world. Dr. Govindan Gopinathan, an accomplished neurologist and a longtime practitioner of Ayurveda, described to me a successful treatment as achieving "a state of balanced humors in the body: a clear soul, regulated emotions, and an engaged mind."

Dr. Gopinathan and I work in the same office building. "It is as if you received the Ayurvedic treatments without actually getting them," he said to me one day as we shared an elevator up to our respective medical offices.

Dr. Gopinathan knows me well. When I fell off my world, he felt my distress. Now he is a witness to my restored equilibrium, to my renewed strength in my physical and spiritual world.

2

The Pulse of Recovery

> People are like stained-glass windows. They
> sparkle and shine when the sun is out, but
> when the darkness sets in their true beauty is
> revealed only if there is light from within.
> —*Elisabeth Kübler-Ross*

The inner pulse can keep beating long after doctors, researchers, and their monitors predict a patient's death. Believing in this essential force can keep you and your family from giving up hope too soon.

In 1985, when I was an intern rotating through the intensive care unit, one of my first patients was a man named James Gould, a forty-year-old restaurant manager and maître d'. Gould had suffered a cardiac arrest and just about died outside the hospital. As is typical for such a sudden and unwitnessed disaster, by the time his heart was brought back, his brain had practically suffocated from lack of oxygen. It's a medical condition known as anoxia. Dr. George Anderson, the neurologist who visited Gould in the ICU, insisted that he would never recover. Yet Anderson couldn't be certain because Gould still had brain function on his EEG, his eyes were still open, and he still responded slightly to pain. "The lights are on, but no one's home," Anderson said, as he wrote his brief, dismissive note in the chart. For some reason, I didn't believe him. Even this early in my training, I accepted the inevitability of progressive sickness and death. I consigned many cases to failure and lack of recovery even before my supervisors did. But something about Gould was different, something I couldn't put my finger on. Even though several weeks passed without a discernible change, I sensed a presence that defied the physical reality—Gould's inner pulse.

As an intern, I tended to disbelieve my own perceptions and my developing intuition, especially when my higher-ups' opinions differed from mine. But Gould was different. I considered him a viable patient, rather than someone in a deep coma with no prospect of regaining a good quality of life who was simply occupying one of our beds until he died.

This was 1985, five years before the Teri Schiavo case first hit the news, and cases like Gould's were quickly dismissed by every doctor involved as unsalvageable. I was appalled when my supervising residents began to mock my continued need to present his case in great detail during daily rounds. There was a convention among residents that the less viable the patient was, the less time an intern spent poring over the details. Very little time was spent examining Gould at his bedside; discussions with the family were avoided entirely, unless they concerned a withdrawal of aggressive medical care; there was a quick consignment of Gould to the circling-the-drain group of patients.

Gould's restaurant was a popular Italian eatery in southern Westchester, and I was able to surmise by speaking with his family that he had been popular there. He was divorced and lived alone, and at first there was no mention of his ex-wife or his child. His sister, a large woman with long, untrimmed blond hair, was his most frequent visitor. She often sat beside his bed for hours. She said she was certain that he could still hear and understand her. She clung to the fact that his heart rate and blood pressure always increased slightly when she came to visit. The notion of Gould being consciously aware inside the hard shell of his unresponsive confinement was infectious—to family members, if not to doctors—and soon more relatives, including his ex-wife and his daughter, visited to see whether his vital signs would increase in their presence, too.

Gould's ex-wife stood two feet from the bed and didn't speak to him or touch him. She was very tall and thin, with large, inexpressive green eyes, which I imagined were still masking the pain of the divorce. Her teenage daughter, on the other hand, came right up to the bed and took her father's limp hand and squeezed it. She stared into his blinking, unsensing eyes as if she were looking into a mirror. She seemed like an incarnation of him, at least physically, with the same dark blue eyes, high forehead, and hair that was so blonde, it was almost white. Her passion for her father was clearly powerful, and I began to wonder whether it was possible that she could help will him back to consciousness. I knew this was an irrational thought, yet I was soon able to elicit a greater response from him. I pinched his nipple, as all doctors-in-training are taught to do, a primitive, yet effective gesture for gauging a pain response, and for the first time in many weeks of similar attempts, this time the maneuver elicited a small groan. "You're hurting him," his daughter objected and glared at me.

"Sorry, but it's a miracle that he can feel pain at all," I replied. "It's a good sign." And it *was* some kind of a miracle. Soon he was twitching his arms and shifting his feet. A day after I reported this finding on rounds and endured sarcastic looks and derisive comments, the nurses confirmed my observations, and all of the doubting Thomases who had previously written Gould off began to

flock to his bedside. He was still mainly a curiosity to these cal-
lous doctors, rather than a viable patient. But then he began to
respond to pain and utter low moans.

My supervising resident now charted Gould's every muscle
twinge or bleep on the monitor and reported them to the critical-
care specialists, as if he'd always believed in Gould's recovery.
Gould's neurologist, Dr. Anderson, who spoke in obscure Latinate
phrases and wore the most expensive-appearing suits and the
shiniest shoes that I'd ever seen in an ICU (and somehow never
got them stained), was now examining Gould several times a day
and proclaiming this the greatest brain recovery he'd ever witnessed in his twenty-five years of practice.

"I always knew he had a chance," he claimed.

What a hypocrite, I thought.

The narrow-minded views of doctors like Anderson were
what kept my profession from acknowledging rare and uncanny
recoveries until they were blatantly obvious. Anderson was one of
the most rigid of them, pompously adherent to his so-called scientific principles. Known as the grab-bag diagnostician, he was
known for making his diagnosis after only a few minutes and then
being unwilling to budge, no matter what further information or
insights surfaced.

A few weeks later, Gould was sitting up in bed and straining
to speak. His voice was high-pitched and squeaky, hoarse from
the many weeks on the respirator, an incongruous sound when
contrasted with his thick chest and large, manly jaw. He began
to speak in sentences of only a few words, subject and verb, but
enough for me to tell that he had maintained his intelligence.
Another neurologist, Dr. Allen, who was covering one weekend
for Anderson, told me that he'd never seen this significant a
recovery from the anoxic encephalopathy (shut off of oxygen to
the brain) that had accompanied Gould's cardiac arrest. Allen, a

gentle old neurologist with soft hands and a large, bald head, was one of the few attending doctors who bothered to speak directly to interns. I could tell that he wasn't a fan of Anderson's.

"When he can speak, ask Mr. Gould what he remembers," Allen said. "Might his drive to survive, combined with his family's support, have helped him recover?" I asked. "Hard to prove," the wise old doctor said. "But I do believe it."

I believe it was his inner pulse. As Gould began to sit up in his bed, his recovery stretched on over several more weeks, and I had him to myself again, as the residents and the attendants forgot about the miracle and focused on what was needed to get him transferred out of the ICU. Now he was simply a slow-thinking, slow-to-speak patient who was taking up a bed. Even when I was a more seasoned physician, I could still never understand this common urge among doctors to free the ICU of patients as soon as they stabilized, when there were many more gains still to be made. Why was the staff so eager to free up his bed when it would instantly be refilled by a patient who required far more work and had much less of a chance to recover?

By not learning from this man's unexpected recovery, a staff wearing blinders would make the same mistakes over and over again and would overlook many unexpected cures. I was searching for something specific that might account for the miracle. As Gould regained his ability to think and reason, I began to ask him what he remembered. He had a memory hole where the last three months should have been. I spoke to him about his near-death experience, but he said he didn't remember anything beyond flashing lights and blurry images. He did recall several out-of-body moments—feeling as if he were looking down at himself from the heart monitor over his bed. Gould told me that he was the kind of person who never gave up, and his entire family reinforced this view. His sister, daughter, and ex-wife all commented on this vital force; they all said they could still feel it even when he was deep in a coma.

His daughter told me that she never doubted that her father would recover. "I could feel it," she said, "long before I could see it." I wondered whether having his daughter and his ex-wife around and feeling their energy had actually helped Gould recover and return from the long deep tunnel of his coma, had enabled him to infuse his pulse with healing energy.

It was clear to me that the divorce from his ex-wife had hit him very hard. She was the first person he asked for when he awoke. He was clearly pleased to hear that she had been coming to see him. He told me that he still hoped to convince her to come back to him. When I first mentioned his daughter, I could see his passion for her in his expression, and I had a stronger view of the love/courage/will that may have enabled him to defy science. Anderson had been ready to pull the plug when the EEG showed minimal upper-brain function, but Gould had defeated the wisdom of the grab-bag neurologist.

Gould is not alone, although his recovery was certainly quite rare. Other recoveries from comas have been even more dramatic. The year before I was an intern treating Gould, in 1984, nineteen-year-old Terry Wallis survived a motor vehicle accident after the pickup truck he was in plunged twenty-five feet into a ravine. He was left paralyzed and comatose for nineteen years before suddenly returning to consciousness one day and blurting out "Mom" when his mother came to visit. Wallis's doctors commented that they believed constant talks from his mother elicited his emotions and helped gradually pull him from his coma. In fact, he awoke on Friday the 13th, nineteen years after the accident, which had also occurred on Friday the 13th.

According to neurological studies, the longer a coma lasts, the less chance a patient has of regaining independent function. When a coma lasts more than a week, the likelihood of achieving a good recovery within a year declines to 7 percent. Patients with a choked-off oxygen supply to the brain (hypoxic or anoxic encephalopathy such as Gould's) have a 58 percent chance of awakening from a coma and a 12 percent chance of making a good recovery. Yet the vast majority of the patients who recover from this kind of coma do so within the first week, and Gould was in his coma for more than three weeks.

In a famous case in 1989, Trisha Meili, jogging in Central Park in New York City, was brutally attacked. She ended up in a coma in the hospital, where Dr. Mary Ann Cohen used a technique on her known as "the running commentary." It was similar to the method that as an intern I had used intuitively with Gould. Dr. Cohen talked to Meili on a daily basis, in the hope that this would establish a connection that would help draw the patient out of her comatose shell. Like me, Dr. Cohen had a deep intuition that her patient would be one of the rare ones to survive. Cohen was quoted in Meili's book *The Central Park Jogger*, "When I first saw you, in a coma and in need of resuscitation, it didn't look good, but my intuition sensed you were going to be fine. I wasn't sure you could get all your mental function back, but I was positive you'd get most of it."

In January 2009 in the UK, a thirty-four-year-old woman named Emma Ray suffered a heart attack and went into a coma nearly two weeks after giving birth. As reported in the *Daily Mail*, she remained in the coma until a kiss from her husband, Andrew, appeared to revive her. Her condition was quite similar to Gould's, in that her brain had been partially starved of needed oxygen (hypoxic encephalopathy). After Emma's two weeks of not responding, Andrew's sudden kiss provoked a return kiss. This was the beginning of a miraculous recovery, which, like Gould's, appeared to be a result of her will to survive and the love of her family.

Paulette Demato, the program coordinator for the Coma Recovery Association, has complained that all too often, families aren't given the opportunity to "wait and see what happens," that the medical community will try to force a family's hand to get them to withdraw treatment from a comatose patient. This was the pressure I felt with Gould, but luckily, he had already begun to recover by the time Anderson was ready to turn off the machines.

I believe Gould's out-of-body experience was an indication of the close tie between his flickering physical life and the larger spiritual world it clung to by his inner pulse. There are many well-known cases of this, perhaps none more famous than the experience of Carl Jung, who wrote about his experience in his autobiography, *Memories, Dreams, and Reflections*:

> It seemed to me that I was high up in space. Far below I saw the globe of the earth, bathed in a gloriously blue light. I saw the deep blue sea and the continents. Far below my feet lay Ceylon, and in the distance ahead of me the subcontinent of India. My field of vision did not include the whole earth, but its global shape was plainly distinguishable and its outlines shone with a silvery gleam through that wonderful blue light. In many places the globe seemed colored, or spotted dark green like oxidized silver. Far away to the left lay a broad expanse—the reddish-yellow desert of Arabia; it was as though the silver of the earth had there assumed a reddish-gold hue.

Then came the Red Sea, and far, far back—as if in the upper left of a map—I could just make out a bit of the Mediterranean. My gaze was directed chiefly toward that. Everything else appeared indistinct. I could also see the snow-covered Himalayas, but in that direction it was foggy or cloudy. I did not look to the right at all. I knew that I was on the point of departing from the earth. Later I discovered how high in space one would have to be to have so extensive a view—approximately a thousand miles!

Jung's out-of-body experience occurred in 1944, but the first satellite photo of the Earth wasn't taken until 1959. Amazingly, Jung's "mental map" conformed to later photos.

Most out-of-body experiences occur while a patient is losing consciousness, often due to exhaustion or physical paralysis. I believe that these experiences demonstrate the mind's connection with the spiritual world, especially when unfettered by the body's usual daily demands.

These experiences and sensations can be reproduced, to some extent. Susan Blackmore, a psychologist in Bristol, England, who herself had an out-of-body experience in the 1970s, was later able to induce these perceptions in subjects by stimulating the temporal lobes of the brain. In 2002, neurologists at Geneva Hospital in Switzerland triggered out-of-body sensations in epileptics by stimulating the angular gyrus of the right cortex of the brain.

In a study published in the August 2007 issue of the journal *Science*, scientists tried to induce out-of-body experiences in healthy people. The research, conducted by neuroscientist Dr. Olaf Blanke at the École Polytechnique Fédérale in Lausanne, was combined with separate experiments carried out by neuroscientist Henrik Ehrson at the Karolinska Institute in Stockholm. Blanke, in his experiments, stroked a fake hand and the subject's real hand simultaneously, until the subject had the sense that the fake hand being stroked was his or her actual hand. Ehrson also used video equipment to allow subjects to see their own backs. He simultaneously stroked a subject's real back while appearing to stroke the image that the person saw. The out-of-body type experience that resulted could be explained by the decoupling of sight and touch. .

Dr. Jeffrey P. Long, a radiation oncologist and a world expert in near-death experiences (NDEs), considers out-of-body experiences to be proof of our inner connections to the spiritual world. "About half of near-death experiences involve a separation of consciousness," Long said to me in an interview. He pointed to the seminal research of Dr. Michael B. Sabon, which showed that those who had a near-death experience following a cardiac arrest had a clear recollection of the details of the resuscitation. Additional research by Janice Holden and others have found an accuracy of recollection of more than 90 percent.

From my own experience and the stories I've uncovered for this book, I believe Long may be right. Near-death experiences can be analyzed by science, but they frequently go beyond it. Long said that people may experience a renewed sense of life from a near-death experience: "Having an NDE is life enhancing. NDErs usually no longer fear death. It gives them courage to live life to the fullest. They become aware that life is purposeful, meaningful; they learn lessons, especially lessons of love. An NDE gives them the will to live and to live with love."

This renewal of the life force seemed to be the case for my patient Gould. Although I hadn't known him before his cardiac arrest, everyone in his family said that he seemed happier and more content after his recovery. After a long stint in the ICU, he was finally transferred out and two weeks later was discharged to go back home. He returned to work at the same restaurant.

The only residual sign that he had of a mild deterioration of mental acuity was that he now worked as a waiter, rather than as maître d' and restaurant manager. Outside the restaurant, he performed better than ever; he saw his daughter far more often, and he once again began to date his ex-wife.

Neither Gould's neurologist Anderson nor his critical-care specialist could explain why he had been spared the usual tragic outcome of an anoxic victim. Why had his brain recovered, when so many other people's brains had not? Had his daughter helped reinfuse him with a life force? A probabilities expert might suggest that Gould was simply the rare case that survived. The vast majority don't recover from this degree of brain injury, but a few, mainly those who have a strong inner pulse, do.

My medical training focused on the pathology of how Gould's brain had strangled without its needed blood and oxygen supply, but this science did not prepare me to consider the power of his emotions and his drive to survive. Yet these intangible forces appeared to be crucial to his recovery.

In medical school, I learned about empirical "facts," the logic of cause and effect, and the world of evidence-based medicine. Penicillin cures a sore throat, blood pressure responds to antihypertensives, surgery removes an infected or a cancerous organ, and people get better. It takes a special kind of learning to consider the effect of the spirit on healing.

Can strong passions directly alter the metabolic potential of the body? The brain, after all, is a soup of chemicals, and in response to the mind's entreaties, the body either speeds up or slows down, sweats, urinates, or dries up like a prune. There is a growing body of medical literature that examines this connection, studies that have begun to show the effect of personality on hormones, emotion on body chemistry, thinking on the actual nerves themselves. Yet no matter how science maps the exact pathways, I believe that the effect of the mind on health goes beyond the physical and verges on the metaphysical. I believe strongly that a powerful intuition-based response may be working to alert a patient long before a test or a finding brings an illness to a doctor's attention. Doctors may also be guided by intuition, but this intuition evolves during a career, as cardiologist Dr. Sandeep Jahuar wrote in the *New York Times*: "When we talk about instinct in medicine, we usually talk about expert clinicians grasping diagnoses in ways that seem to defy analytical explanation. These doctors appear to know almost intuitively which data to focus on and which to ignore. Of course, their decision-making is based on experience and deductive reasoning (and perhaps on evidence, too), yet it seems almost mystical."

This doctorly intuition may grow from a direct connection with patients' intuition, creating an inner pulse radar. Unfortunately, this kind of connection seems to be rarer than ever before. Overdependence on tests and their growing precision has lulled many a doctor such as Anderson into a false sense of security that blunts instinct. One antidote for this kind of reductionist thinking is to be found in the patient's story itself. Narratives introduce quirky, yet illustrative examples that cut against the grain of medical mantras. For Gould, it was the day-to-day narrative that added up to recovery. The monitor continued to beep on, and each day revealed a patient who was slightly more responsive than the day before. The days accumulated until a miracle was finally acknowledged by all. Anne Harrington believes that the power of suggestion has a great capacity to heal and to maintain "a powerful hold on the contemporary imagination." Today's doctors tend to place too much stock on direct physical evidence. We doctors, as well as our patients, need a more expansive way of thinking that includes an emotional and intuitive narrative that our patients can relate to.

Too many patients are frustrated by a medical system in which test results are the primary focus, answers are often impersonal, and emotions are disregarded. Patients are in revolt these days against such attempts to write them off too soon, to peg them into pre-decided diseases and prognoses based on the symptoms of disease alone.

Their rebellion is justified. The solution is to broaden our perspective, to consider the emotional, as well as the physical, and to examine the spiritual tie that binds them together. Many sick patients know when they are going to die or perhaps survive against the odds before any test or doctor-messenger tells them. We can all learn from this knowledge.

Recovery may be predicted when a patient or a healer has a galvanizing moment that is infused with a deep perception of the inner pulse.

3

One Patient, Many Pulses

Dissociative identity disorder can result when a child with an unstable identity is subject to severe emotional trauma over an extended period of time.

—Dr. Richard P. Kluft, Temple University

The inner pulse is the power that holds the body and the soul together. Gaining access to this great power may even allow you to affect a disease as seemingly incurable as diabetes.

When I first graduated from my medical residency and started in private practice in the early 1990s, I was grateful for all new patients, as many young "hungry" internists are. I was soon known for being easily accessible. I could be called on for a last-minute medical clearance for surgery, for electroconvulsive therapy, or for any patient who developed an unexpected medical problem.

When I first met Connie Jones, I had no idea who had sent her to my office. She was wearing thick glasses and a faded yellow skirt and blouse. She was slight, just over five feet tall, reserved, and timid.

"I am here for my diabetes," she said matter-of-factly.

"Is anything bothering you?" I asked, trying to elicit what doctors call a patient's "chief complaint."

Connie seemed startled by the question. "Nothing. Nothing at all," she said.

"What can I do for you today?" I asked, but instead of answering, Connie showed me her blood glucose meter, the handheld machine that measures blood sugar levels. She suddenly pricked her finger with the tiny metal lancet and squeezed out the single drop of blood necessary for an accurate glucose reading. By that measure, her glucose level—the amount of sugar in her blood—was within the normal range.

Connie denied tingling feet, thirst, or blurry vision, the common symptoms of a poorly managed diabetic condition. Strangely, despite her knowledge about her condition, she denied having had regular visits with another internist or endocrinologist before seeing me. She said she could take care of her diabetes herself and that she had been injecting a single shot of insulin a day for several months. When I asked Connie where she had obtained the medication, she explained, again without apparent emotion, "I am a registered nurse at St. Mary's Hospital in Queens. A doctor I work with prescribes my insulin for me." I found it difficult to believe that any doctor would prescribe insulin without seeing her as a patient, but I couldn't tell at this point what the truth was.

The science of diabetes is clear: patients lack an adequate ability to absorb glucose from the blood into their cells, either because they don't secrete enough insulin, a hormone made by the pancreas, or because they don't respond to the insulin they do make. With type 1 diabetes, often called juvenile diabetes, the primary problem lies with the pancreas; with type 2, often called adult-onset diabetes though it is occurring in younger people because of the current obesity epidemic, the main problem is resistance to insulin. In either case, prolonged exposure to high blood sugar levels can cause circulatory problems and nerve damage. These circulatory problems cause sluggish blood flow in the legs and abnormalities in the retinas of the eyes.

Yet my examination turned up none of these telltale signs of diabetes. Connie's foot pulses and retinas were normal, and the soles of her feet were normally sensitive to the prick of a pin.

I thought that perhaps Connie lacked the typical signs of diabetes-related damage because, at thirty-nine, she may not have been diabetic for very long. I suspected she had a variety of type 2 diabetes that required insulin. Back in the 1990s when Connie came to see me, however, before long-acting Lantus insulin was developed, a single-shot daily insulin regimen was usually inadequate. Most patients needed more.

After I drew Connie's blood, I wrote out a prescription for two shots per day. I said that I would increase the complexity and frequency of her shots when I was sure she could manage them. Connie promised to check her glucose level throughout the day and give me a list of the results. She was strangely nonchalant about her diabetes, but she did seem ready to follow my directions. She agreed that I would be the doctor prescribing her insulin from now on, and she scheduled an appointment for the following week.

When Connie didn't show up for the appointment, my office manager at the time, Mona, called her. She made another appointment, but Connie skipped that one, too.

"Who referred this patient to me in the first place?" I asked Mona. This was a question that I, young and hungry for patients, didn't always bother to ask in those days.

"No one," she replied. "She walked in off the street."

I couldn't call the hospital where Connie said she worked—it would be a violation of her privacy—and I had no other way to check on the truth of her story. I decided to wait. Her first blood tests had come back fine. Her glucose was normal, which wasn't that unusual for a diabetic (they often vary during the day), but I was more interested in the results of her hemoglobin AIC, or glycosylated hemoglobin. This is a measurement of the amount of sugar that adheres to red blood cells, and it is initially elevated in many diabetes patients, then returns to a normal range with treatment. Connie's number, 5.6, could have been the result of a well-treated case of diabetes, or it could have indicated someone who had never had diabetes at all. It occurred to me that I had no objective evidence that Connie really was diabetic besides her statement, and she certainly didn't seem to be very reliable.

The next time I saw her, she arrived without an appointment, so changed in appearance that I didn't recognize her. She was wearing shorts, a ripped T-shirt, and a red fedora, and her face was streaked with smeared makeup. She cursed at Mona, who recognized her before I did and asked me what to do. I suggested that we draw blood for a drug toxicology screen, as well as for glucose. Under the bright lights of the examining room, Connie became polite and cordial again. The drug screen was normal, but her glucose level was now 250 milligrams per deciliter of blood. Depending on when a person last ate, the normal glucose level can range from 70 to 110.

Here was the objective evidence I needed that Connie really was diabetic. I was unhappy with myself for doubting her. I wondered whether she had been complying with my instructions for her insulin. Her careless dress and attention-seeking behavior didn't suggest compliance, although she continued to say that she could handle a complex daily treatment regimen consisting of several insulin injections of varying amounts. "I know how to handle my diabetes," she insisted. "I'm a nurse."

I reluctantly designed a more elaborate insulin schedule for her because she insisted on it. If she followed my outlined schedule, the amount of insulin she took would depend on her blood sugar readings on the glucose meter.

The following day I tried to call Connie at her hospital (I had gotten her permission to do so). I didn't reach her, but to my relief, her supervisor confirmed that Connie did indeed work there. She offered that although Connie was a little strange, she was a good nurse. She also volunteered that Connie was diabetic and denied that she got her insulin from any of the hospital's doctors.

A week after showing up in the fedora, Connie called. She said that she was following my orders closely and that her blood sugar levels were normal.

At the time of Connie's next appointment, a patient appeared at the front desk dressed in a mannish blue suit. Although Mona recognized the patient as Connie, the patient insisted on filling out a new patient information form. Mona brought me the completed form with a puzzled look. The address, the phone number, and the other information were exactly the same as Connie's, except that the patient listed his name as "Donald," his age as twenty-two, and his diagnosis as unknown.

In the examining room, I asked Connie whether she was taking her insulin.

"My name is Donald," she replied, "and I am not a diabetic."

I asked Donald whether he felt stressed. When he nodded, I gently asked whether he would consider seeing a psychiatrist. Donald said he didn't think he needed to see one. I explained that he might find it helpful to talk about what was making him feel so stressed. After I gave him my reasons, he agreed to go. He didn't need much convincing, although he denied having seen a psychiatrist previously. I referred him to Dr. Ralph Spicer, an astute evaluator of severe mental illness who had recently completed his training.

I suspected that Connie could be suffering from dissociative identity disorder, then known as multiple personality disorder, a condition that—despite its media popularity—is actually quite rare. After evaluating Connie, Dr. Spicer called me and said he had discovered that Connie had actually been in treatment for this problem for many years with a different psychiatrist. I relayed to Spicer my concern that Connie's disorder could be interfering with her management of her diabetes. Her blood sugar levels seemed to vary, depending on the personality she was manifesting. I didn't yet accept the wild, unprecedented idea that she could affect her blood sugar directly, based on the hormonal force of one personality over another. I suspected instead that one personality (known as an "alter") would comply with the treatment and keep her blood sugar levels stable, but another alter would disregard the regimen, and her levels would swing out of control.

"Well, you'll have a chance to test your theory," Spicer said. "I'm not sure if her sugars are out of control, but her personalities certainly are. I'm admitting her to the hospital."

In the hospital, my initial theory was proved wrong. The nurses on the psychiatric ward watched Connie carefully. The head nurse made sure that Connie's blood glucose levels and food intake were checked and recorded around the clock. There was little chance for noncompliance. Nevertheless, Connie's glucose level frequently rose out of control and then dropped back down to normal.

Another wilder idea occurred to me. Could the inner pulse, the life force that bounded with good health and waned to faintness with severe illness, be fragmented? Could Connie have a different spiritual force depending on which personality was active? Could each inner force have a profoundly different effect on her or his metabolism, leading to decidedly different blood glucose levels? Connie was now undergoing intensive psychotherapy, and as she cycled from one personality to the next, the psychiatric nurses documented significant swings in her glucose levels.

One of Connie's alters was "Phyllis," a placid sixty-year-old former schoolteacher who was apparently very sensitive to insulin. On one particular day, Phyllis's glucose level was 52. Forty minutes later, Phyllis claimed to be Connie. Connie, who tended to be moody, had a glucose level of 185. The alter named "Tamara," who seemed to be the ill-mannered young woman I had encountered wearing the fedora, had a glucose level of 212. Yet the alter named "Rachel," a twelve-year-old girl who liked to wear flowery dresses and loathed taking any kind of medicine, had a glucose level that never exceeded 100. Most of the time, in fact, Rachel refused to take her insulin, claiming that she wasn't diabetic, and the nurses had to wait for another personality to emerge before giving it to her.

During the two months that Connie was in the hospital, the psychiatric nurses documented more than forty personalities—all with distinctive voices, postures, and temperaments. Donald, who had the cracking tenor of an adolescent boy, was calm and stood very straight. Tamara, a nervous chain-smoker, had a shrill voice. Rachel's voice was soft and sweet; Rachel never smoked and was never upset. They all had different baseline blood sugar levels.

I was unable to prove that the fluctuations in Connie's blood sugar were directly caused by changes of personality or by a change in the inner pulse warping the body's physical and hormonal responses, but it was difficult to explain things any other way. There was a clear link between how upset she was and her blood sugar level, which strongly hinted that the level was associated with the hormonal response. In addition, none of the alters who claimed to be diabetes-free were ever found to have a glucose level higher than 150, whereas the alters of Connie, Tamara, and "Shirley"—a self-described jazz singer who walked with a pronounced limp—often did.

Dr. Spicer never pinpointed the exact onset of Connie's psychiatric problems, but he learned from her prior psychiatrist that she had had dissociative identity disorder for many years in a much milder form, where the differences among the alters were more subtle. Ultimately, Spicer settled on Connie as the core personality, and the staff began to work on helping her integrate the other personalities. For medical reasons, I was disappointed. Connie was not the alter with the best glucose levels. She was a nurse who knew about diabetes, but her glucose levels varied greatly.

The identity of Connie also didn't seem to me to be the best choice from a psychiatric point of view, although it wasn't my place to say so. At one point in her hospitalization, Connie ordered Donald to kill himself and threatened to send a gun to him. That murderous intent eventually dissolved, and Spicer thought that she was ready to go home. The nurses disagreed, but Spicer discharged Connie anyway. He wrote in her discharge note that her personality shifts were much less frequent and milder.

Spicer was right, at least at first. By the time she was involved with a violent struggle that led to her untimely death, I hadn't seen her in many months.

But right after leaving the hospital, Connie did surprisingly well. She was compliant with a complex treatment regimen of five insulin injections a day, and she kept her appointments with Spicer and with me. She managed to hold on to her job as a nurse. Her employer decided not to pursue the matter of how she had actually obtained her insulin before coming to me.

There is a growing body of medical literature that reveals the effects of positive emotions and spirit on the ability to fight off infection, hasten wound healing, and improve overall physical functioning. On the detrimental side, stress and negative emotions have been shown to speed the heart rate, raise blood

pressure, increase metabolic function, and heighten susceptibility to infection. It has also been shown that personality can
directly affect bodily functions, and that certain conditions, such
as irritable bowel syndrome and fibromyalgia, are strongly related
to highly stressed personality types.

As far as I can tell, Connie's case is unique. With Connie, the
extremes of her personality and the switches in her inner pulse
appeared to affect her physiology to such an extreme extent that
her basic metabolic function was altered. She knew this truth
about herself long before her doctors did; it was up to us to catch
up. As I matured as a physician, it was becoming more and more
clear to me that medical science provided us with a far too narrow definition of disease and cure.

I will never know the origins of Connie's psychiatric problems. What I do know is that she was diabetic, at least as Connie.
Yet the condition of her other alters raises fascinating questions
about whether the mind can overcome its usual constraints to
the point that it can alter basic glucose metabolism. Can diabetes result directly from the mind's effect on the body? Was this
patient's personality essentially dictating the type of hormonal
and receptor-organ response that defined her as diabetic? Could
Donald, who claimed to be diabetes-free, have remained healthy
without receiving any insulin for the rest of his life? Could
Phyllis? I don't really think so, but sometimes I do wonder.

Dissociative identity disorder is frequently misunderstood,
misdiagnosed, and even mocked. Yet the primary diagnostic textbook of psychiatry (DSM IV-TR) takes it seriously, defining it as

A) the presence of two or more distinct identities or per-
     sonality states, each with its own relatively enduring
     pattern of perceiving, relating to, and thinking about
     the environment and self;

B) at least two of these identities recurrently take control of the person's behavior; and

C) inability to recall important personal information that is too extensive to be explained by ordinary forgetfulness.

Taking my lead from the textbook, I accepted that Connie suffered from this extraordinary condition. The notion of different personalities each taking control of the person's behavior was a description of dueling inner pulses, each with its own psychic foundation.

Dissociative identity disorder, or DID, supposedly results when a child with an unstable identity encounters severe emotional trauma during an extended period of time. The child eventually creates new identities with which to hide from memories, explained Dr. Richard P. Kluft, a clinical professor of psychiatry at Temple University and a psychiatric consultant for Showtime's series *The United States of Tara*. A February 2009 Canadian study in *Nature Neuroscience* showed that early childhood trauma could change the hormonal and stress responses in the brain and predispose certain patients toward DID.

Dr. Richard J. Loewenstein, the medical director of the Trauma Disorders Program at the Shephard Pratt Health System in Baltimore and, like Kluft, a world expert on DID, said that the differences between alters are generally subtler than Connie's. Yet "florid differences do sometimes occur," Lowenstein acknowledged, "and may be associated with a much poorer prognosis."

Kluft argued that the disorder can sometimes be faked. Dr. Richard Van Dyck, a dissociative-identity expert and an emeritus professor of psychiatry at VU University Medical Center in Amsterdam, said that it's difficult to "differentiate true dissociative cases from simulated cases."

Not all psychiatric experts believe that the disorder really even exists, contended Dr. Jess P. Shatkin, the director of education and training at the NYU Child Study Center. "During my career, I've only seen one convincing case," he said, "and even then I think that some of the seventeen identified 'personalities' were fabricated."

Research on DID indicates that alternate personalities—if they do exist—vary widely and may cross gender lines, and that alters such as Connie, Donald, and others may have a varying level of awareness of one another.

Studies have confirmed metabolic differences between the personalities in a patient with dissociative identity disorder. Blood pressure, heart rate, and even the EEGs that measure electrical activity in the brain vary from one personality to the next.

What about blood sugar? This important chemical has never been directly examined to see how it varies depending on personality type, or how it may vary from personality to personality in a patient with DID. Yet there is a scientific basis for believing that it does. The amount of sugar in our blood is determined by a complex interaction of several hormones, which changes when we are frightened or upset. In a stressful situation, the amygdala in the brain triggers a hormonal response known as fight or flight. Receptors in the neck and the adrenal glands—small glands that sit on top of the kidneys—release hormones that prepare the body to react.

This fight-or-flight reaction provokes us to break down sugar we have stored in our tissue. The sugar floods into the bloodstream, giving us the energy we need to respond quickly to a threat. At the same time, more insulin is produced by the pancreas, enabling us to use the sugar and store the excess. A person with diabetes such as Connie, however, either can't make the amount of insulin she needs to help use the blood sugar, or can't properly absorb it into the tissues. The result is a persistent elevation in sugar. Although the blood is flooded with sugar, the muscles are still starving for this fuel.

Kluft said to me that he has treated hundreds of cases of DID with various physiological (body activity) findings. He has observed the activation of different brain functions in different states of mind, with different manifestations of the inner pulse in each case. Kluft indicated that the brain patterns for DID, also described by researcher Bruce Perry, are in sharp contrast to the typical higher-brain function associated with normal thinking. According to Kluft, stress-related states such as DID show less blood flow to the frontal areas and more activity in the amygdala, the fear and emotional center of the brain. Consider that these states of stress are associated with increased levels of epinephrine, norepinephrine, glucagon, and cortisol, the very hormones that lead to increased glucose production. This could certainly explain why Connie's shift from one personality to the next was often accompanied by rising sugar levels in the blood. Loewenstein has noted variable heart rate and blood pressure associated with switches from one alter to the next, "with heart rate literally falling by 50% in one case immediately after a switch." Loewenstein agreed with Kluft that shifts in personality "are accompanied by major psychobiological changes, usually related to activation of the brain's HPA [hypothalmus-pituitary-adrenal] axis. . . . One can certainly hypothesize that blood sugar is among the variables that change related to different behavioral states."

According to Loewenstein, if the patient becomes acutely anxious, blood sugar will rise; if she freezes in her tracks, incapable of escape, blood glucose will drop. Kluft agreed, saying that he had treated a patient with insulin-dependent diabetes like Connie who could raise or drop her glucose 50–150 milligrams per deciliter merely with a switch of personalities. "If she slipped into an alternate personality with a freeze response [where she became immobile], the sugar tended to drop," Kluft said. "If it was a fright response and she ran, the blood sugar soared. I saw her drop to a normal blood sugar level within an hour after hypnotic/psycho-therapeutic interventions. I saw a normal blood sugar skyrocket when an unexpected spontaneous recalling of a traumatic event occurred and restabilize when the reaction was finished."

Despite these dramatic examples, the jury is still out on the exact relationship between glucose and personality, though it is clear that a strong correlation does exist. What was most uncanny and unprecedented in Connie's case were the ways that her different alters were able to control hormones and maintain their respective glucose levels.

The notion that one's personality can determine one's blood sugar level defies traditional science. There are no cases exactly like Connie's in the medical literature, in part because the kind of mind control she exhibited is extremely rare. Yet less extreme examples are found in the world every day. When our blood sugar is low, we are upset or anxious. Hormones are released to cause our blood sugars to rise, and then when the levels are high enough, we are able to exhibit more self-control. These routine occurrences are driven by our inner pulse's need to achieve equilibrium.

Connie's inner pulse was fractured and flailing. Connie's healing involved restoring the unity of her inner pulse, at least temporarily. Once consolidation occurred, Connie was reunified, with all of her personalities living in one body. She was diabetic all of the time now, with her newly fused inner pulse better at eliciting her nursing skills than it was at stimulating her pancreas to produce insulin.

Unfortunately for diabetic Connie, this inner pulse fusion did not last.

4

Inner Pulse Rising

> The cradle rocks above an abyss, and common sense tells us that our existence is but a brief crack of light between two eternities of darkness.
>
> —*Vladimir Nabokov*

The inner pulse is not linear; it does not follow a predictable path. It ebbs and flows like a current. Because this central life force is ever changing, these changes are not easy to perceive, and a weakening in the pulse can suddenly strengthen and vice versa—this is one reason that both health and illness are never entirely predictable for even the most discerning patients or their doctors.

Recovery is often characterized by almost imperceptible increments; the same is true for the fading of the inner pulse with worsening illness. Sometimes the pulse is snuffed out all at once by a tragic accident, while at other times it gradually diminishes, one part of the body at a time. Sometimes the inner pulse has more power left to it than a patient or a doctor knows.

Sensing a slowing of the inner pulse can be misleading. It can cause a patient to give up too soon, to count himself out before his time. Yet sometimes a patient with conviction realizes that his inner pulse is still stronger than others perceive it to be. A patient may reach for an inner strength that no one else believed he still had, which emanates from the pulse. He may run a race that no one thought he could still run or solve a puzzle that no longer seemed solvable.

The inner pulse may surge, for one final glorious moment, and enable a patient who is paralyzed to walk again.

In the ultra-hot summer of 1997, just two weeks after the birth of our first child following a difficult pregnancy, my tall, dark, Russian-born wife, Luda, was given a choice: either give up her long-coveted fellowship in neurophysiology at the university or return to work there immediately. Her supervisor, an old-fashioned Eastern European doctor, was insistant, so back to work she went, filled with a fresh appreciation for the suffering of her patients.

One patient who immediately benefited from Luda's heightened empathy was Brian Solomon. As Luda completed her fellowship and took the first tentative steps into the world of private practice, she supplemented her income by working Wednesday afternoons at the Muscular Dystrophy Clinic. Brian Solomon was a seventy-year-old man with severe muscle weakness from a muscle-destroying inflammation known as inclusion body myositis. Solomon was a regular at the clinic, and he quickly grew to love my wife's easy manner. He was soon calling her Luda and asking her to transfer him away from the clinic to her fledgling private practice. Luda was careful not to rob the clinic of its patients, but she made an exception in Brian's case, telling me it was because of his warmth and familiarity. "He's like an old uncle of mine," she said, and she admitted a special sensitivity for his growing weakness. Luda's mother spent her days in a wheelchair from the debilitating effects of multiple sclerosis.

My wife and I shared office space, and I soon came to know many of her patients. Brian introduced himself to me one day in the fall of 1998 as I was walking through Luda's waiting room.

"Marc," he said, and I stopped, surprised by the stranger's familiarity. I scrutinized this man in the wheelchair—his legs and arms were visibly atrophied, yet were covered with thick bristles of hair that seemed to suggest a more active man. His neck was thick, and his head was covered with downy white hair that reminded me of my grandmother. His jowly face was the only body part where constant activity still remained—his eyes were roving and hyper-alert.

I soon felt comfortable around Brian, too. He requested that I be his internist, and he would wheel across the hall to my exam rooms just after he'd visited my wife. She was treating his affliction with intravenous gamma globulin, following the well-studied theory that his disease was autoimmune. He was making antibodies to his muscles that caused the inclusion bodies to form and crowd out vibrant strands of muscle fiber. The IVIG, as it was known, blocked the antibodies the body made against itself before these antibodies could do more damage.

Both Brian and my wife felt that his treatment was working. He didn't tolerate it very well from my internist's perspective, often developing high blood pressure or heart failure when he received it, but he looked forward to these three-day stints of intravenous therapy in the hospital. He regained pockets of strength in his arms and legs for months afterward.

Even before Brian told me his big secret, I could sense that he was an angry man. The sorry details of his fractured life gradually became apparent to me during several hospital and office visits.

It took so much effort for Brian to come to see us, maneuvering weakly from his apartment to the access-a-ride ambulette to the office service elevator to my waiting room, that I felt guilty limiting our conversations to the few chronic medical issues he had—high blood pressure and high cholesterol. Instead, I found myself listening for many minutes to the specific details of his unhappiness.

He was divorced from his first wife, who had left him for the family accountant. Brian had lost access to his only son, Rob, during the ugly legal battle, but when his ex-wife decided that she wanted a freer lifestyle, Brian had raised Rob from his early teens. This should have endeared the boy to Brian, but Brian said that Rob continued to blame him for the divorce. When Rob got married and had children himself, Brian was rarely invited over to see them.

When Brian first got sick, Rob would call my wife monthly for updates, but I met him only once, during a period when Brian was severely depressed and refusing all treatments. Rob, a tall unshaven man with poor posture, came to my office and demanded that his father be admitted to the psychiatric ward of our hospital. I declined, because in my opinion, although Brian was clearly depressed and needed a psychiatrist, he was not a threat to himself, and he was refusing hospital admission. Rob didn't call me after this, and I never saw him again during Brian's visits.

Brian saw himself as a kind of lawyer, although he said he had never been to law school. During one of his IVIG treatments in August 1999, I recall sitting in a chair in Brian's room on the seventeenth floor of our hospital as the sun streamed in the window and obscured his facial expressions. The intravenous gamma globulin dripped into his veins while he revealed his secret to me.

"Roger Lefferts was a personal injury lawyer in Brooklyn," Brian began. "Ten years ago I was hired to be his clerk. I didn't know any formal law, but he was lazy, and I was motivated and quick thinking in those days, so he began turning a lot of the case work over to me. I read the law books at night, researched the relevant statutes, and soon I was solving his cases for him."

"Did you ever think of going to law school?" I asked him.

"Many times. But I couldn't afford it."

"Didn't he pay you for solving his cases for him?"

"We made an arrangement. I was supposed to get 20 percent. He paid me a little. Claimed he was cash poor. That he would pay me later. After twelve years he owed me more than two million dollars. But I had nothing in writing."

"*Two million*! Was this a legal business?"

Brian laughed weakly, full of the memory of what his life had been. "Does it sound strictly legal to you?"

"Were you afraid that if you tried to report him for not paying you that you could go to jail yourself for being involved with him and knowing that some of his cases weren't strictly legal?"

"Yes, of course."

"Why did you stay with him?" I asked.

"I kept thinking he would pay me, and I had nowhere else to go to work. Finally, I got too weak to keep working." Brian sighed, his eyes glazing over with the memory. "As I got sicker, I began to think of how much more medical care I could afford if only I had the money he owed me. After a while, I could think of nothing else. I called him. Begged him for it. At first he said he would pay me, but then he stopped taking my calls."

"Can you forget about it now? It doesn't sound like you have much chance of collecting at this point," I said sensibly.

"I can't forget it. I dream of it, of confronting him for his money. Every time I can't get out of the wheelchair or am unable to get myself to bed or I almost fall off the toilet, I think of him in his beautiful house with his fancy cars and maids and kids in private schools and I think, This guy doesn't deserve to live." Brian gritted his teeth and spoke in a low rasp. "If I could get his money by rising out of my wheelchair and killing him, I would do it. I swear I would. I dream of it."

As his doctor, I was concerned that the anger and the intent were real. As fond as I was of Brian, nevertheless I now ignored his refusal and called a psychiatrist to see him. When the psychiatrist, Dr. Jeff Goldberg, a soft-spoken, rather unkempt man, came to his room, Brian suddenly decided to talk. Goldberg had a way of making his patients feel comfortable, in part because he looked a bit like a patient himself. Yet I knew him to have a razor-sharp set of psychiatric skills. Afterward, he called me and said he wasn't concerned. "It's a lifelong obsession with this former boss. I think it's real and not delusional. It fuels itself, but overall, I think it's harmless. His plan always involves him rising out of his wheelchair to attack. Since he can no longer physically do that, it's a sign of a pure fantasy. If he had a plan that was actually possible, like hiring a hit man, I'd be more concerned."

I was more concerned than Goldberg was. I had a strong intuition that Solomon was to be taken seriously, but I also trusted Goldberg's opinion, despite his depraved appearance, and felt that he was rarely wrong. Nevertheless, when Brian refused the antidepressants Goldberg prescribed and continued to say that his only pleasure in life would be to see his former boss dead, I decided to call in a second opinion.

This psychiatrist, Dr. Andrei Topalov, a jovial Bulgarian former Olympic wrestling champion, was more concerned. We discussed Brian in the hallway outside his room. "This is homicidal rage," he said. "Luckily for us, he doesn't have a plan that will work, and he isn't capable of making this happen."

"You mean, he doesn't have the right kind of connections," I said.

"Exactly," Topalov said, with a short, uncomfortable laugh. "And getting out of his wheelchair to do it himself is impossible. Nonsense."

I wasn't so sure that Topalov was right.

Brian Solomon had married for the second time in the late 1970s, and his new wife, Louise, was not healthy either. They had settled in a small ranch house on a half acre of property in North Babylon, Long Island, which Brian proudly described as lined with hundred-year-old poplar trees. Brian stared out his hospital window at the East River and longed to return home, imagining a certain armchair lounger or a particular view from his paneled den out to his back yard.

Louise, however, was often reluctant to take Brian back. My wife and I had had many phone calls with Louise, in which we reassured her that Brian was stable enough to come back from the hospital after a bad bout of pneumonia or "fluid overload" following an intravenous gamma globulin treatment. His inner pulse was fading but was still strong enough to sustain him.

These calls became more frequent as Brian became weaker in 1999 and early 2000. When I first knew him, I used to anticipate his walker-aided marches through my office, but these had been replaced by his wheeling in by wheelchair. By late 1999, Brian had qualified for Medicaid, and he was able to hire an aide, a quiet African American man named Felix. Felix had a good sense of humor and laughed at Brian's jokes, and he began to wheel Brian everywhere. He was supposed to work eight hours but often worked closer to twelve. He soon took over the main caretaker role from Louise. Louise, a former social worker in the Babylon school system, continued to display her ambivalence at receiving Brian back after a hospital stay. I sensed that Brian's frequent bursts of anger, combined with his worsening disability, drove her to the point of desperation.

Yet it was also clear to me that Brian adored and relied on Louise. I'm sure it was painful to Brian that he couldn't provide better for her. He surely blamed Lefferts. He had told me of his dreams to outfit his house with the equipment and the staff that they needed to care for both of them, if only Lefferts had paid what was owed. The house still had a few years left on its original mortgage, and they were living on Louise's small pension, plus social security and the few thousand dollars that Brian had saved. When Brian spoke of his hatred of Lefferts, he was referring not only to the comfort care that he had lost, but also to Louise's discomfort. She was a survivor of throat cancer, and she spoke in a thin rasp created by a mechanical speaking device. She had a failing heart and was frequently short of breath.

As Brian got weaker, Louise was the first to speak of nursing homes. The sicker they both became, the more Brian talked about seeking revenge on Lefferts. Brian confided in me that his deepest intuition informed him that he still possessed the strength in his body to rise up out of his wheelchair one more time to attack Lefferts and claim what he was owed. Brian dreamed frequently of this moment, and he also insisted that it was within his power to make it happen. Such a possibility went well beyond the scientific reality of his illness, but Brian said he was sure that he could do it.

If the hospital psychiatrists had known of the inner pulse—if they had been familiar with its manifestations—they might have taken Brian's proclamations more seriously.

Of course, the inner pulse is not strictly measurable, but I had the sense that Brian's inner pulse was still stronger than any doctor might guess by looking at his physical appearance. When

I closed my eyes and imagined Brian, it was a man striding forward, not collapsed and weak in his wheelchair.

One night in the summer of 1999, long after Felix had gone
home for the night, Louise phoned me at one o'clock in the
morning to say that Brian had fallen off his lounger. Louise had
tried to help him but had developed chest pain herself and was
now lying on the floor, trying to catch her breath. "I can't take this
anymore," she rasped. "He has to go. I want a divorce."

I called 911 and sent an ambulance to the house. They were
both taken to a local hospital, and although Louise was soon
released, she managed to convince the hospital staff to place
Brian in a local nursing home.

I thought he would never return home after that. I thought his
inner pulse was really fading this time, but again he proved me
wrong by recovering. He even managed to talk Louise into taking
him back one more time, and by the fall he was once again taking the small access-a-ride ambulette to my office. "Got any jokes
to tell?" he would ask me whenever he rolled in, and I knew he
would have an assortment ready by the time I had examined him,
and he had wheeled to my consultation room for a chat. Humor
was another sign that his inner pulse was still beating, because
dying patients rarely tell jokes. Yet along with his humor, Brian
continued to have bursts of anger mixed with periods of depression, and he grew even weaker.

"Have you spoken to Rob lately?" I often asked him, and
although he always said yes, behind his head his trusty aide Felix
indicated no to me with his eyes.

"Louise and Rob don't get along," the aide informed me when
Brian was having his blood drawn in another room by my nurse.
"Rob says that Louise is mean to Brian, and Louise says that Rob
is worthless."

Felix wasn't the first nurse's aide to carefully map out the family dynamics even as he tended to a patient's bodily needs.

"Rob's using Louise as an excuse," I said. "He should be there. Brian was there for him when his mother abandoned him. Brian brought him up and was a devoted parent to his son."

Felix slowly nodded his agreement. Apparently he knew this story, too. Brian was a man of great heart, in my experience another common feature of a strong inner pulse that refuses to die.

Early on the morning of September 21, 2000, Brian Solomon asked Felix to drive him to an address in Brooklyn. Felix didn't find this request particularly unusual. Brian had told Felix that he had once worked in the law offices at that address, and one of his customary activities during the last few months was to be driven to this neighborhood. A few weeks earlier, Felix had parked the Toyota minivan and lowered Brian into his motorized wheelchair, and as they sat in a café across the street from 185 Montague, Brian had stared silently for hours. Felix couldn't tell me whether Brian recognized anyone coming in or out of the building, but he later commented to me that during the next few weeks, Brian's gaze had seemed to grow more intense. Felix had ascribed this to Brian's growing anxiety, rather than to anything specific, although it was clear to me that his inner pulse was getting stronger.

Felix later remarked to me that on this September day, Brian's mind was focused elsewhere. "He seemed to almost be in some kind of a trance," Felix said. So Felix gave his patient the benefit of the doubt. Like Brian's doctors, Felix was too quick to dismiss Brian's growing mental focus and resolve. His inner pulse was pounding, but no one was noticing.

I blamed myself afterward for not accepting Brian's intuition as a warning that he could accomplish this and for not taking definitive action to restrain him. Brian's inner pulse was focusing, and soon he might be able to draw more power from it to overcome his physical limitations. It was Brian's case that finally convinced me to act on my patients' instincts and sense of their inner pulses, even when it seemed to defy science. It wasn't until afterward that I could really visualize Brian, the paralegal, sitting in Lefferts's office and solving case after case for him while receiving no pay up front. After the tragic event, I could finally see the psychic friction building toward combustion, as each tangible but unaffordable health need was contrasted with the ledger he had kept listing his personal accounts receivable for cases solved. When Felix rolled the wheelchair out of the van on Montague that fateful morning, the point of action had been reached, a fulcrum where the inner pulse engaged the muscles.

Miraculously, Brian wheeled himself to Lefferts's office, lifted himself up and out of the wheelchair without assistance, pulled out a gun, and shot Lefferts. Brian's muscles were so atrophied that he was able to lift his arm only high enough to shoot Lefferts in the foot, so Lefferts survived.

Here's how the *New York Times* reported it:

Witnesses heard the two men arguing and then heard a gunshot, the police said. Mr. Solomon apparently fired twice, first missing the lawyer and then hitting him in the leg with the second shot.

Afterward, Brian told the police that he was suffering from chest pain. He was taken to Long Island College Hospital in Queens, instead of immediately to jail. A stunned Lefferts was brought to St. Vincent's Hospital on the West Side of Manhattan, where the bullet was quickly removed and he was reported to be in stable condition. Brian was soon released from the hospital and brought to jail and, as the *New York Times* reported it, charged with attempted murder, first-degree assault, and criminal possession of a weapon. I am not sure whether my wife, Luda, was his one permitted phone call, but she told me that Brian had called and said that Louise and Rob would not speak to him and had refused to post bail.

Brian's attorney contacted us a few days later to file an affidavit attesting to his inability to serve a prison term, due to his disability and profound weakness. We were both glad to do this, confirming that Brian was wheelchair bound and suffered from a profound progressive muscle disease, and that the events of September 21 were an aberration due to some kind of emotion-driven metabolic frenzy that temporarily reinvigorated his inner pulse.

The judge accepted our explanation, and Brian was released, having served only three weeks of his fifteen-year sentence. Afterward, he returned to my office to see me, making jokes as if nothing had happened. He seemed relieved. His obsessive fixation with Lefferts had gone. The failed shooting had provided an emotional, as well as a physical, release.

Brian's inner pulse had allowed him to overcome his physical limits and rise like an enraged animal to attack.

Emotion channeled through his inner pulse had trumped scientific prediction. Afterward, he slumped back down into his wheelchair as his life force ebbed once again.

After the shooting, Louise no longer allowed him to come home. The house in North Babylon was in her name, and she was so outraged by the crime that she flatly refused to take him back. I called her several times, but she would not relent, claiming that she was now afraid that he would physically harm her, too.

After his next admission to the hospital for gamma globulin treatments, Brian had nowhere to go, and the social worker had to arrange for a nursing home for him. I managed to get him admitted to the Cardinal Cooke facility in Manhattan, where he said he enjoyed the irony of being a Jew in a church-run home.

His visits to our offices dropped off after that, ostensibly because of logistical difficulties in arranging the ambulette from Cardinal Cooke. When I did see him, I could sense that his inner pulse was fading; he wasn't measurably sicker or weaker, but I could just tell that he was losing his hold on life as he became more withdrawn. A year after the shooting, I heard from Brian's son, Rob, that Brian had died. The official cause was a progressive muscle-wasting disease.

The inner pulse has control over our bodies and our minds and can produce a trance or hypnosis, states of intense concentration. Hypnosis is accompanied by a decrease of peripheral awareness and potentially improved and enhanced performance skills. It is likely that Brian was in a trancelike state as he approached Montague Street.

Trance can be quite powerful, according to Harvard researcher Dr. Martin Orne: "If we incorporate our psyche within the realm of our conscious, we can attain a higher level of spirituality, peace, and enable our mentality to overcome physical and mental weaknesses. Practicing trance concentration through our psyche, we capacitate ourselves with unimaginable forces of nature." Trance is a manifestation of the inner pulse. With trance the individual retains awareness of what he is doing, and with hypnosis he does not.

When I asked Brian about what had happened afterward, he freely recounted much of the event, which suggests trance. Yet he also appeared to enter a state of hypnosis as he approached Lefferts that fateful day on Montague Street. Hypnosis shows the power of a focused inner pulse and has been defined as the ability to "help us transcend or rise above what physically is happening in order to begin changing that physical experience."

There are many mythical and historical examples pertaining to superhuman strength and trance. In the Bible, Samson entered a state of super-concentration and overcame the Philistines with strength that derived from his hair and God and a strong inner pulse, and the mythical heroes Achilles and Hercules used their strength to subdue their opponents. Historically, the Berserkers were Norse warriors who were known for their fearless strength and immunity to pain.

There have been several well-known examples that demonstrate the channeling of the inner pulse into super-strength in an emergency. On September 11, 2001, in the midst of the World Trade Center catastrophe, a group of people lifted a heavy cabinet off a coworker who was stuck underneath it. A firsthand account puts it this way: "One of my coworkers, Frances, was in the Xerox room and was almost crushed by one of the cabinets. In a matter of seconds we were all in the room trying to lift the cabinets and open the exit door enough so that we could crawl through. It's true what they say about superhuman strength when the adrenaline is running. We finally did it."

The sudden physiological surge can be described as excited delirium syndrome. The patient's sympathetic nervous system shifts into overdrive, and excess amounts of the vessel-constricting, heart-thumping hormones adrenaline, noradrenaline, and cortisol are released. The heart speeds up and pumps harder, the nerves fire more quickly, more glucose is made, the skin cools down and gets goose bumps, the eyes dilate to see better, and blood flow increases to the vital organs, including the brain, the liver, and the kidneys. The message is received by the brain that it is time to do something.

British physiologist Gavin Sandercock concluded in his research that there is a neuromuscular reserve in untrained individuals that can be tapped into in extreme circumstances as a result of the "turning off of the negative feedback from mechano receptors in the muscle and particularly Golgi tendon organs." Exercise expert Lindsay Edwards, in his work, also supported the notion that there may be a protective mechanism in the brain that keeps us from having access to our superhuman strength except in the most dire circumstances. Under great stress, the emotional center of the brain takes over.

Scientist David Behm, a professor of philosophy and rehabilitation science at Memorial University of Newfoundland, found differences among individuals and among various muscle groups. In a study, he found that the quadriceps were under the most inhibition from the brain.

Only a sudden surge from the inner pulse could explain Solomon's unexpected ability to rise out of his wheelchair that fateful day. Back in 1961, Michio Ikai and Arthur Steinhaus of George Williams College, in a classic study published in the *Journal of Applied Physiology*, discovered that when it came to "performing muscles," "acquired inhibitions" could be overcome by disinhibition.

The workings of the inner pulse defy simple explanation. The pulse is the place where the powers of the mind and the body come together. Dualists, beginning with Descartes, have argued that the mind can affect the physical world through direct control of the body. Sudden super-strength is an extreme example of this mind-body effect.

5

Radar to Die

All interest in disease and death is only another expression of interest in life.

—*Thomas Mann*

Sometimes a patient can believe he is dying when he isn't. This kind of foreboding, sadly, can become a self-fulfilling prophecy.

Jim Lambert caught my attention because he offered me a free gift in the middle of my busy office one Monday in the spring of 2002. Some of my patients knew how to pull strings—medicine is so demanding of a doctor's emotions that anyone who brings an office staff donuts or flowers or brings a doctor a bottle of liquor instantly gets our attention. Lambert was even more generous than most; this sixty-six-year-old owner of a limousine company immediately offered to give me free limo rides anywhere I wanted to go.

I soon discovered that Lambert was fearful of doctors and hoped that his offer would engage me in a superstitious back and forth that would somehow keep bad things from happening to him. I decided not to compromise our professional relationship by accepting his free limousine rides.

It was difficult to convince him to remove his clothes or to sit on the table when he sat in my examination room for the first time. He jumped around, nervously waving his arms. He had a mop of gray hair and an unshaven pointed chin, and the large veins in his neck stood out like plumbing pipes as he gesticulated. His raspy voice was the result of what he admitted was a three-pack-per-day smoking history over several years.

"I hate doctors," he told me. "Can't stand 'em. All they have is bad news. If I avoid going to them, I figure I can live longer."

"Why are you here?"

"I called your hospital. They recommended you. But I doubt it will last."

"I'm not going to push you into anything," I said, as gently as I could. Like Lambert, I am high strung, and he was already making me nervous. "You'll decide what you're comfortable with. I just want to examine you."

He leaned back against the examination table but did not climb up onto it, and he still would not remove his clothes. In this position, I was at least able to examine his heart and lungs and take his blood pressure, which was much higher than normal, at 180/105. When I suggested the possibility of a pill to lower his blood pressure, he refused. When I placed my index finger on his wrist to take his pulse, he jerked back. "I just want to check your heart rate," I said.

"We both know it's racing," he replied.

"Why are you so nervous?" I asked.

We moved to my consultation room. He looked out the window and fidgeted on my blue fake leather couch, a movement that caused a high-pitched squeaking sound and probably made him even more anxious. Sitting there, he confided that he had been avoiding doctors for the last five years, ever since an internist had ordered a CT scan of his lungs and the report mentioned a possibility of cancer. Instead of repeating the scan in a few months, as the doctor had suggested, Lambert had run away. He said he was constantly worried that he was going to start to cough up blood and die.

He removed a soiled, matted piece of paper from his back pocket and handed it to me across the desk. As I opened it, I saw that it was the CT scan report. It described a 2-centimeter noncalcified nodule and suggested a biopsy or a repeat scan, neither of which Lambert had had. For five years he had lived with an almost palpable fear of cancer while continuing to smoke at the same rate. It had never occurred to him that these five years of having no symptoms other than his usual smoker's cough suggested that the nodule wasn't malignant—if it were, he would surely be dead by now or at least be coughing up blood.

"Many of those suspicious nodules never develop into anything," I said aloud. "You've outlived the significance of this CT scan, which is great news. I'd like to do another one, but only as a precaution."

Lambert decided on the spot to allow my positive reassuring attitude to push him into the long-dreaded scan. He ran from my office right to the CT scanner at the medical center three blocks away. A few hours later, we knew for certain that the nodule hadn't changed in five years, and there were no other suspicious nodules.

When I called him on his cell phone with the good news, I expected him to be relieved and show some emotion, but he simply said thanks and hung up the phone. I tried to call back, but his cell phone went straight to voice mail.

He missed his follow-up appointment a week later, and it took my office nurse several phone calls and messages before she could persuade him to come back in.

When I examined him this time, his blood pressure was even higher than before, 190/110, and although this pressure probably wasn't life threatening, it certainly demanded treatment. I tried to talk with him about it as he squeaked on the blue couch, but he would only say that revisiting the CT scan issue and removing the report from his back pocket had triggered a new set of jitters that now seemed to be unstoppable. It occurred to me that Lambert's fear of death had been focused on the CT scan report, which, although it was ominous, also held the possibility of a reprieve. Now that the reprieve had been given, he was back to free-floating dread.

It appeared that deep worry was an essential part of his personality. Worry was his negative radar. He was a deeply rooted mass of nervous symptoms looking for a cause to attach itself to.

Lambert told me that he was now worried that he would have a stroke. I decided to use this as leverage to convince him to take blood pressure medication, which would lessen his risks dramatically. But he said he was afraid of the side effects of the medicine, and I found it difficult to convince him that the risk of a stroke was far greater. Even as he continued to refuse treatment, however, he kept coming to see me.

After another visit to my office, with his blood pressure in a perilously high range of 190/115, he finally agreed to take a beta blocker, a medicine that directly relaxed and slowed the heart, while dilating the blood vessels. This would be the perfect treatment for him—it often had the side effect of making patients calmer.

He agreed to take the medicine, and when I saw him a week later, his blood pressure had come down to a more reasonable 150/85. He said he was still anxious much of the time, but he wouldn't take medicine for anxiety, and he wouldn't see a psychiatrist.

"What are you so anxious about?" I asked him.

"I'm going to die, I just know it," he said fatalistically.

Anxiety plays a role in provoking high blood pressure by causing the body to release stress hormones (epinephrine and norepinephrine) that constrict the blood vessels. The beta blocker interfered with this mechanism.

"You are not going to die," I said. "You don't have lung cancer, and we are getting your blood pressure under control. Your risks of a sudden emergency are reducing dramatically."

"You are a good doctor," he said. "But I know I am going to die."

Lambert told me that when he was most panicked, he forgot to take his blood pressure medicine. I urged him to institute a routine of morning pill taking that would disarm his premonitions. Eventually, however, on one of his most anxious days, with his pill bottle unopened, his blood pressure rose out of control, and he developed a sudden excruciating headache and blurry vision. By the time the paramedics arrived at his house, his blood pressure was 220/120.

In the ambulance he became unresponsive, and his eye pupils constricted to pinpoints. The paramedics could tell that he was experiencing a sudden bleed into his head. They put an endotracheal tube down his throat into his trachea, breathing for him as rapidly as possible in order to blow off carbon dioxide and try to reduce the swelling in his brain—but it was too late. By the time the ambulance reached the hospital, Lambert was dead.

I've gone over this case many times in my mind, and I continue to wonder what I might have done differently to improve poor Jim's compliance and get him treated for his anxiety while there was still time. In retrospect, of course, I wish I had accepted his premonition more and not been so dismissive of it. At the same time that his raw fear was provoking the very hormones that would do him in, this same fear was also his warning system—his connection to the inner pulse—that something dreadful was about to happen.

Despite all of the situations I'd had where the patient's instincts had been right and the science had been wrong, somehow I had ignored the signs in Lambert's case. I was too eager to perceive intuition as positive and too quick to dismiss dread as simple panic. Dread is an important radar in its own right, a warning system that must be paid attention to. Even when science predicts life, a patient's inner pulse can predict death.

After Lambert's death, I was a different doctor. I was much more responsive to my patients' negative intuition and much quicker to follow the path of their unease, even when science didn't predict what it was they were most afraid of.

Premonitions of death are not always as straightforward as Lambert's. When the inner pulse weakens, it is not always the patient who is aware of it. Sometimes it is a loved one, and, clouded by his or her own emotions, this relative may not always have the most accurate insights. A premonition that someone is about to die or that the inner pulse is about to extinguish may be misdirected. I recall a startling case where a daughter was in contact with her parents' inner pulse and felt that severe illness and death were near, but she was convinced that it was her mother who was dying when it was really her father. She sensed a weakening of the inner pulse but had the wrong pulse.

A few years ago, when my eighty-two-year-old stroke patient Phyllis Silverstein came to my office, her daughter Hannah, rather than her usual aide, was pushing her wheelchair. "Something's wrong with my mother," she said.

Hannah lived in Israel, and I'd never met her before. She continued without introduction, "She's losing weight. I feel she is going to die. I want her to come back to Israel with me."

I examined Phyllis more closely than usual but still found nothing wrong. She weighed seven pounds less than she had a year earlier. A diabetic, she had suffered frequent infections of her toes, but she had none now. She was joking and friendly with me the way she always was, and I was tempted to believe that the real issue with Hannah was that she wanted her mother and father to live near her. Hannah's father, Rabbi Mordecai Silverstein, formerly the head of the largest synagogue in Newark, was already ninety-one.

Yet I took Hannah's premonition seriously because of her strong conviction that her mother's inner pulse was fatally fading, so I put her mother through a strenuous work-up of CT scans for her weight loss and a colonoscopy, tests that all came back negative. When I saw Phyllis a month later, she seemed more vital than before and hadn't lost any additional weight, which was a good sign.

Still, her daughter wasn't convinced, so I worried. My experience with Lambert had convinced me that a patient's or, in this case, a family's premonition could be directly connected to the inner pulse in a way that could be stronger than my own developing medical intuition. I called Phyllis on the phone frequently and scheduled her for monthly visits. Her daughter returned to Israel and did her worrying from a distance of several thousand miles.

Rabbi Mordecai Silverstein had been a close associate of Lubavitcher Rebbe Rabbi Menachem Schneerson. By the time of his death in the 1990s, Schneerson had taken on almost mythical significance as a Jewish prophet. Rabbi Silverstein had often been his emissary on trips around the world on behalf of Jewish interests. Silverstein had been the rabbi of one of New Jersey's main Orthodox synagogues for many years; people from all over the city came to him for help. I knew he cared greatly for his wife, yet during her admissions for stroke, infections, and even toe amputations, he had never sounded anxious or worried. He spoke in a slow, measured voice, and his eyes quickly glimmered in response to a perceived irony or joke.

Even at age ninety-one, Rabbi Silverstein still liked to drive. Since he wasn't my patient, I couldn't know whether he was still capable of it. His wife had often suggested that he come to see me for a physical, but he said he was happy with his own physician, who had been following him for many years. In what would turn out to be one of his final mitzvahs, the great rabbi called an Orthodox Jewish school in New York and recommended my three-year-old Sam for admission to the nursery.

On the morning of Wednesday, March 5, Silverstein drove to Jersey City from Manhattan to appear with his son Saul on his celebrated Jewish morning radio program. It was a special program, commemorating twenty-five years on the air. Mordecai said on the air that he was very proud of his son.

Driving back alone afterward, according to Phyllis, old Mordecai was apparently trying to avoid traffic on the Pulaski Skyway and chose to take Duncan Avenue, which dead-ends into the Hackensack River, underneath the skyway. As reported in the New York Times, cars had gone into the river off Duncan Avenue several times in the past. The road was wet that day, so the rabbi may have skidded, or else he may have fallen asleep at the wheel after a tiring morning, but in either case, his car, an old Ford, was discovered in the river two days later. There was no sign of foul play.

I called Phyllis on the phone when I heard of Mordecai's sudden death. She sounded strong—her inner pulse bounding.

All of her children and several of her grandchildren were with her, and her four sons were flying their father's body to Israel for burial right after Shabbat.

I visited Phyllis in her home that Sunday, a visit to surviving relatives known as a shiva call, and she looked surprisingly resilient and calm. She didn't appear to have lost more weight, even through the process of intense grieving. Hundreds of religious Jews from all over New York had come to pay their respects to Mordecai. Yet Phyllis took the time to sit with my young daughter, Rebecca, and speak softly to her about her love for drawing and painting. Phyllis was strong and thriving, even as her husband lost his inner pulse and died.

Hannah's premonition that one of her parents wasn't going to make it back to Israel alive had been correct, although she had chosen the wrong parent. A premonition is still a premonition, even if the aim is off. By premonition, I mean a strong intuitive sense that there is about to be a shift in the inner pulse, a significant weakening and even death.

Hannah's feeling of disquiet over her mother's health was a prophecy of her father's death. She had sensed it, had known it was about to happen, but perhaps her emotions had interfered with her intuitive radar. She knew the inner pulse was weakening in someone close to her; she was simply wrong about who it was. Still, I didn't believe Hannah's sudden concerns, which were soon followed by her father's death, were a coincidence, just as Lambert's premonitory dread had been connected directly to his death.

Premonitions are often sensory experiences that range from gut feelings or uneasiness to actual hallucinations. The sensation that something is about to happen may be tied to disasters, deaths, or other emotionally charged events. These feelings of uneasiness emanate from the inner pulse. It is the pulse—the nexus connecting the life force with the greater spiritual world—that weakens dramatically when death is imminent. A premonition as I define it is a sense that the inner pulse is starting to change, right before it manifests this change physically.

There are many startling historical accounts of premonitions. In 1948, the Soviet psychic Wolf Messing was in Ashkhabad when he reportedly felt dread. He sensed that a pervasive weakening of the life force was building throughout the city. He canceled his performances for the only time in his life and left the city. Three days later, a massive earthquake hit Ashkhabad, killing fifty thousand.

The *Titanic* carried only slightly more than half of its passenger load on its sole voyage in April 1912. The psychiatrist Ian Stevenson recorded several incidents of premonitions concerning the *Titanic* in England, America, Canada, and Brazil in the two weeks prior to the sailing. Some people canceled their reservations after reportedly dreaming of the disaster.

A patient's advanced warning system is a dramatic manifestation of his inner pulse. The patient may sense that his inner pulse or those around him is beginning to weaken, and he may respond viscerally to this foreknowledge.

In 1966, a landslide of coal waste buried a school in Aberfan, Wales, and killed 116 children and 28 adults. This landslide was preceded by hundreds of cases in the town of premonitions and precognitions (which included choking sensations and seeing black clouds). A deeply intuitive person may feel the massive internal rumble of a town's inner pulse about to be snuffed out.

There were many stories of people who missed the fateful flights of 9/11 because of premonitions. All four of the hijacked planes were carrying only half the usual number of passengers, in part because of cancellations. Can sudden shifts in the inner pulse that cause patients to experience premonitions be mea-sured indirectly? Psychologist Dean Radin, a senior scientist at the Institute of Noetic Sciences, worked on the U.S. military's Stargate program, where he hooked up volunteers to a machine that measured electrical currents across the skin. Subjects reacted to seeing violent or threatening videos. Radin found that people began to react a few seconds in advance of the image, even though there was no warning signal that the image would appear.

Other researchers in Scotland and at Cornell University in the United States duplicated these results. Dick Bierman, a psychologist at the University of Amsterdam, used a functional MRI scanner (which measures increased blood flow to areas of the brain with increased activity) to examine the brain's reaction to the images from Radin's experiments. He concluded that the brain was going through verifiable changes in anticipation of star-tling events, just as the inner pulse began to change.

It isn't only people who have these kinds of premonitions. There are also stories of animals that are in touch with their own-ers' inner pulse and react strongly when death is near and the pulse is fading fast. In the *New England Journal of Medicine* in July 2007, Dr. David M. Dosa, a geriatrician at Brown University, described Oscar the Cat, whose bedside visits to the residents of a nursing home in Providence, Rhode Island, were an indica-tion of impending death. I spoke with Dr. Dosa in early 2010 on the publication of his book *Making Rounds with Oscar*, which describes their professional experiences together visiting patients at the nursing home. Dosa agreed that Oscar was sensing the final weakening and stopping of the inner pulse of the dying patients. Dosa said that fifty patients who died during the last four years had received visits from Oscar the week before their deaths. Oscar was rarely wrong. His appearance in a patient's room was always an ominous sign.

"Oscar is not a friendly cat," Dosa said.

I asked Dosa what he thought was the secret of Oscar's special skill to sense the weakening of a patient's inner pulse.

Dosa, a pleasant geriatrician with a calm manner, said he thought that many more animals probably had this skill. "I think it's connected to the sense of smell. Pheromones, or some kind of biological odor that people and animals give off when they are about to die and their inner pulse, as you call it, is stopping."

According to Dr. Dosa, Oscar's death watch never kicked in with enough time to save the patient. Yet although Oscar sensed only the final death throes of the inner pulse as that crucial vital sign was extinguished, this skill was useful. Oscar's alert did give families a chance to plan for their loved ones' deaths and to come in to say good-bye before their relatives died.

Though the inner pulse defies direct measurement, I was learning more about how I could be guided by its shifts. As it waxes and wanes, strengthens and fades, it predicts the future. The inner pulse predicts whether we are going to live or die, and it may give us time to prepare for both the evitable and the inevitable.

PART TWO

The Healing Pulse

Three quarters of the miseries and misunder-
standings in the world would finish if people
were to put on the shoes of their adversaries
and understood their points of view.

—*Mahatma Gandhi*

6

Dancing in the Dark

He who knows others is learned; he who knows himself is wise.

—*Lao-Tzu*

Physicians often mistake the real signs of illness because we rely too much on our textbook-driven expectations. I was learning a different way, a way to complement the textbook. This way cannot be measured, it is not strictly reproducible, but I was learning how to recognize it. It was becoming part of my method of healing, as well as part of my spiritual worldview. It focused on the inner pulse as our personal connection to a greater reality. The more I learned about the inner pulse, the more my patients benefited.

It was difficult for the hospital's psychiatrists to find internists who were willing to enter the locked doors of our hospital's psychiatric ward. As a young internist in the early 1990s, I was one who would.

One patient, Kim Bradley, claimed to have a strong intuition about her health that her doctors were overlooking. She was a twenty-five-year-old singer-songwriter who had been admitted to the hospital's psychiatric ward with the diagnosis of bipolar disorder, in the throes of a manic rage. When I went to see her one blustery fall day in 1993, however, she seemed calm and rational. I was there to perform a basic medical evaluation.

Kim became anxious when I began to examine her neck, feeling for the tip of her thyroid, just below the Adam's apple. "There's something in my neck, I know it," she said breathlessly. "No one can find it." Kim held her hands in front of her neck with a gesture of self-protection. Her room smelled of sweat. I had asked her roommate to leave so that I could examine Kim privately, but the roommate had refused, so I was examining Kim behind a thin curtain hastily drawn around her bed. I could sense her roommate staring through the curtain at us. Kim was thin, though not to the point of being emaciated. I could smell the cigarette smoke on her breath, and I could see its effects on her yellow fingernails. She had straight red hair, and she had tied it behind her neck with a rubber band. She stared at me intensely, and I realized that she could probably erupt into screams at any time.

I knew that psychiatrists were sometimes blatantly wrong in their diagnoses. More than once, I had been asked to provide medical clearance for a depressed patient to receive electroconvulsive (shock) therapy, only to find the patient unexpectedly conversational. I worried and wondered in these cases whether I should take a role in blocking the shock procedure if I didn't think it was warranted. Though I was an internist, not a psychiatrist, I didn't feel comfortable just rubber-stamping procedures that might not be indicated. Yet I didn't say anything. I knew that I was often fooled. Sometimes the structure of a psych ward made a patient seem more normal than he or she really was. Sometimes a very anxious patient was simply trying to get me to be her advocate by acting calm and solicitous, reminiscent of the way the paranoid patient approached his physician in Chekhov's story "Ward Six."

When I examined Kim's neck, the source of her worry, I wasn't trying to gauge her emotional reactions, I was looking for her thyroid gland. Normal glands are undetectable. You can feel the thyroid protrude from within its bony enclave of ribbed bones in the neck only if the gland is pathologically enlarged.

Like all physicians, I was adept at some parts of a physical examination and poor at other parts. The heart and the lungs were my strengths. I could hear the slightest murmuring swoosh of a leaky heart valve, as well as the tiniest sandpapery sound of a congested lung. I was less confident when examining thyroids. I knew I often missed the bobbing tip beneath a swath of neck muscles. For me to discover a protruberance in the neck, it had to be large. When my probing fingers bumped up against the tip of Kim's thyroid in her lower neck, I knew that I had found a deranged gland. I returned to the nurses' station and checked the computer to see whether thyroid function tests had been ordered—they hadn't. I entered these orders and added a test for thyroid antibodies, which often accompany cases of an inflamed thyroid.

While I was reading through her chart, the psychiatrist in charge of the ward, Dr. John Blum, approached me. I had known John for many years. He was an expert diagnostician, and although he sometimes lacked compassion for his patients, I had found that he was usually good at treating them. John viewed psychiatry as a 9-to-5 job, and his thinking during these hours was goal-directed. He was an effective administrator for this reason, even if the residents and the nurses under his supervision complained that he didn't really care.

John was tall, thin, and blond, a well-muscled, young-for-a-boss psychiatrist. He was gay and out, and he spent a lot of his free time socializing and working out in the gym.

"I'm glad you're checking her thyroid," John said, standing next to me as I wrote my note in Kim's chart, "but I don't expect it's playing a major role here. This is a woman who thinks she's occupied by demons. If I didn't think she was floridly manic, I might have called in an exorcist."

"Hyperthyroidism can cause mania," I insisted.

John smiled. He enjoyed a challenge from a colleague. "Look, Marc. She was attacked in an alley at the age of fourteen. You're not going to find this in her chart, but she was gang raped and choked, left to die on the frozen ground. Somehow she was able to crawl out of there and was rescued, spending weeks in a coma afterward. She's been preoccupied with her neck ever since. Who can blame her? When she's psychotic, she feels as if she's chok-ing. This is not her thyroid, this is Kim being Kim."

The "who can blame her" was uncharacteristic for John. It was clear that he cared for this patient. She was human to him, a victim he wanted to help. "But you're underestimating the effect of an out-of-whack thyroid," I told him. I recalled another patient of mine, Jesse, a thirty-four-year-old man who slept ten hours a day and was exhausted for the remaining fourteen hours. His physical examination and laboratory results had all been nor-mal, with one exception: a thyroid stimulating hormone level of 6.3, which was slightly high, a sign that the tiny peanut-shaped pituitary gland in the brain had been working overtime to push the thyroid gland to make thyroid hormone. The normal TSH range is between 1 and 8 but closer to 1. The higher the number, the more pushing an underperforming thyroid needs. This man had the kind of results that were often not treated, but because he was tired, listless, and constipated (another sign of a poorly functioning thyroid), I'd decided to treat him with a low dose of Synthroid, a human thyroid-replacement hormone.

My treatment regimen was intuitive, certainly not textbook, but the results were staggering. In three weeks, the patient reported a tremendous improvement in his energy. He was soon requiring only seven hours of sleep per night. Whereas before he drank four cups of coffee each day just to keep working, he was down to one cup a day. He now reported having sex with his wife once a day, rather than once every other week.

"Those stories are few and far between," John said. "Much more common is the patient who takes Synthroid and feels no different."

"We'll see," I said.

I was looking at Kim's lab results on the computer screen. John was still standing close to me, leaning into my personal space in a way that you might not expect a psychiatric expert in personal boundaries to do. All at once, I discovered the key medication; in addition to her antipsychotics and antidepressants and antianxiety agents, Kim was already taking Synthroid! Human thyroid replacement hormone is not really a medication, I reassured many reluctant patients, Synthroid is a substitute for what your body is supposed to be making. John said that Kim had initially refused the pill, claiming that it was poisoning her, but then the staff of nurses had simply included it with the assortment of pills that she was compelled to take.

Sitting by the computer, smelling John's pleasantly minted breath near me, I knew instinctively that he was wrong about Kim. For John, Kim's preoccupation with her neck was entirely psychotic—if he asked her, she would say that she was occupied by demons. It all stemmed from the attack in the alley so many years earlier. Yet for me, her neck preoccupation was a strong intuition—despite all of her anxiety—that she still knew herself better than John did. Her inner pulse was signaling her that something wasn't right in her body. I had felt the edge of her thyroid—it was inflamed. This was a hot fact. Whereas I was slowly learning to trust the intuition of my patients, John was moving in another direction: adhering to his diagnosis once he had it. He was often brilliant, often right, but not one to consider a change of course once he'd enacted an entire treatment plan that depended on his being right.

John preferred to have his plan continue, even though Kim wasn't improving, and she was crying out for a change. It would have been wise for John to look for alternate approaches, but although he'd consulted me on Kim's case, he hadn't yet really considered what I was saying. Her racing heart, her sweating forehead, her warm skin—for John, all of these symptoms were still psychosis.

John left as soon as I turned away from the computer screen and began to write my note in Kim's chart. He knew that as a consultant, I was entitled to my opinion, and he trusted me to take charge of her medical issues. I ordered Kim's thyroid laboratory tests repeated. I would have to wait three days for the results. In the meantime, John grudgingly allowed me to stop Kim's Synthroid, which I believed would cause an immediate improvement. Whereas my patient Jesse needed the Synthroid, Kim probably didn't. John didn't agree but acknowledged that the thyroid treatment was my domain. I believed that she had Graves' disease—her body was making antibodies against her thyroid that caused the gland to overproduce. I believed Synthroid (which may have been started before the Graves' disease began) compounded the problem by adding even more thyroid hormone, much more than her body needed, which revved up her metabolism and sent her into an escalating state of mania.

After writing a note in Kim's chart, I decided to return to her room before leaving the ward. I wanted to recheck her thyroid gland one more time. The Kim I found in room 1015 seemed to be psychotic. She was screaming and moaning before she saw me. Her hair was matted to her head by what could just have easily been the sweat from panic, rather than a metabolic disorder. It wasn't easy for a doctor to tell the difference. When she saw me, she immediately grabbed for her neck, and I thought she was going to try to choke herself. There was simply no way I would be able to examine her again that day.

"Monster!" she screamed at me. "Carrion picker! White-coated demon!"

Not wanting to give up, I took a step toward her, but again she reflexively covered her neck with her hands as if she expected me to assault her. By the time a nurse and a security guard came to the room, Kim was up on her bed, shouting in a low voice and banging the walls with her hands.

"She's possessed," Curtis, the burly security guard, said. Curtis was a mixture of large amounts of both fat and muscle. Despite an enormous belly, he seemed *Cuckoo's Nest* strong, and he wrapped his large arms around Kim and lifted her off the bed. The nurse, Alice, a thin woman who seemed more appropriate for a radiology suite than an out-of-control psych ward, held a syringe of antipsychotic medication in her shaky hands. I didn't think she was going to risk jabbing the syringe at a moving target. The security guard was going to have to formally restrain Kim first.

Alice nodded in agreement at Curtis's diagnosis, which differed dramatically from John's or mine. "I've only seen this degree of demonic possession one time before. It took repeated dousing with holy water before she calmed down even slightly." Alice said that she was a devout Catholic who believed in possession and exorcism. John would call the whole episode "hysteria." Not having gone through formal psychoanalysis, John nevertheless loved to speculate on what Freud might have said.

Contemporary treatments for Kim's condition—in John's view—didn't involve Freudian psychoanalysis but instead relied on mood-stabilizing medications such as Depakote or Lamictal. When patients removed their clothes and used their beds as podiums for their rants, heavy antipsychotic medications were added to gain therapeutic control. John was an astute psychiatrist and had a solid understanding of most of his patients' conditions, but with Kim Bradley, he was proved wrong. The angry edge of the gland I'd felt was confirmed by ultrasound, and her TSH level was very low, less than .01, because the pituitary in the brain (hormonal Grand Central Station) was suppressed by too much thyroid hormone in the body (a feedback loop that told the pituitary that the thyroid needed no stimulating).

Her thyroid gland was roaring, producing far more thyroid hormone than the body could use, and the last thing that Kim needed was the additional thyroid hormone in the form of the Synthroid that the psychiatrists were giving her. Her body's own antibodies had turned against the thyroid, attaching to its receptors and causing it to make more and more hormone. As the gland went into overdrive, it grew bigger to accommodate the demand, like a factory with a big increase in customer orders, and now it was enlarged to the point where even my fumbling fingers could detect it in her neck. Kim had sensed it, intuited it, long before any science had caught up and detected it. Her inner pulse had directed her, and I was the first physician to sense it, too. She knew something was wrong, had known it for months, but she was being routinely discounted and her opinions dismissed.

Graves' disease is the most common form of hyperthyroidism, which affects eight times more women than men. It clearly should have been diagnosed far earlier in Kim's case, but it had been overlooked. Luckily, it was a treatable condition. Her chart indicated that she was refusing all new medical treatments, yet she now readily drank the radioactive iodine we ordered to destroy the overactive thyroid cells. She seemed to understand instinctively that this treatment was battling her real disease, and as her thyroid shrunk back to normal size in her neck, she began to report that she was feeling better. She quickly became calmer. An endocrinologist would have to watch her condition closely, because the treatment for Graves' disease often threw the thyroid into a low-producing state, and then she would once again have to take thyroid replacement hormone, Synthroid. Only this time she would actually need it. I had a feeling that she would then welcome it.

When I came to see her in the psych ward on the day of her discharge to go home, she was no longer covered in sweat. Her red hair was lustrous and recently washed, and it was tied back neatly behind her shoulder. She was dressed in jeans and a dark blue shirt and sat calmly on her bed without moving. "How is your neck?" I asked.

"My neck?" Now that her neck was treated, it was clear that she was no longer preoccupied with it. Her thinking seemed calm and clear. The change was dramatic. She was still taking a small amount of Depakote, but her other psych meds had been stopped as her mania receded with the shrinking thyroid.

"Thank you, Doctor," she said, sounding unsure about what she was thanking me for, although it was clear that she was aware I'd played a role.

Kim was a successful blues singer and songwriter. Her band would keep her busy in the studio and the late-night club when she was once again healthy enough to work. I thought she was almost ready.

"Are you returning to your music?"

"Yes, I'm planning to."

She seemed eager, yet subdued, and I was suddenly concerned that my treatment—which had removed her wild rage—could also cost her some of her creativity. Should I have considered her musical talent before ordering the treatment?

A creative personality is a complex mixture of traits. Had the radioactive iodine that Kim gladly drunk to cure her raging neck also diminished her songwriter's spirit? Kim evidently didn't think so. She told me that she couldn't wait to write songs again. She said she felt more in control as a result of the treatment.

Time would tell how fast her inner pulse was really meant to beat. Did the center of Kim's creative impulses lie in a fast-thinking brain, a rapidly beating heart, or the deranged cauliflower-shaped gland in her neck that was now quietly subdued?

Interpretations of the inner pulse and its manifestations depend entirely on perspective. For some it is religious, for others it is mystical, and for still others it represents a sophisticated science that has yet to be discovered.

Kim's nurse considered her "possessed by demons." A century earlier, this would have been the prevailing thought and would have dictated the approach and the treatment. Studying the cultural landscape of "possession" in the 1960s, anthropologist Erika Bourguignon found that 74 percent of almost five hundred societies told stories about possession and that half of them had ceremonies for treating it. Anne Harrington, in her book *The Cure Within*, wrote that "every culture shapes its experiences of possession in accordance with its own beliefs, institutions, and social structure."

Notions of possession and exorcism trace back to our earliest religions. More than three thousand years ago, records of Jewish societies described a belief in demons that were capable of entering bodies and causing them to become ill, although the afflicted people were completely curable by prayer. Christian gospels also wrote of Jesus casting out demons in his role as a healer.

In the Middle Ages, the Catholic Church set a policy that only priests could perform exorcisms. At the same time, societal forces of skepticism and reformation were moving against the exorcism movement. In 1598, when King Henry IV famously asked the physician Michel Marescot to investigate a case of seeming possession, Marescot—a skeptic—gave the young girl consecrated water but told her it was plain water, and nothing happened. Conversely, when he had excerpts from the *Aenid* read to her and pretended that they were from the Bible, she responded with convulsions, a clear sign that she probably suffered from what would be known today as conversion hysteria, rather than demonic possession.

In the eighteenth century, German exorcist Father Johann Larryph Gassner encountered another skeptic, the physician Franz Anton Mesmer, who believed that it was magnetism, rather than demons, that caused violent convulsions. For Mesmer, the so-called convulsions—probably not actual seizures—were part of the cure, rather than due to any demonic affliction.

By the nineteenth century, science was gaining ground, and obsessions with magnetic forces were being replaced by an increasing interest in hypnotism that didn't rely on animal magnetism. In 1882, in a landmark lecture before the French Academy of Sciences, neurologist Jean-Martin Charcot suggested that hypnosis could be produced only in patients suffering from hysteria. Yet a rival of Charcot's, internal medicine doctor Hippolyte Bernheim, believed that suggestibility was natural to all human beings and that hysteria could be both reproduced and relieved by suggestion. Bernheim discounted Charcot by pointing out that he had nothing to say about how the brain or the nervous system really worked.

It took a neurologist in the late nineteenth century to put the work of both men together into a new revolutionary system of thinking about the human psyche and how it could break down in hysteria and be treatable by a new kind of hypnosis. This neurologist was the grandmaster of modern psychiatry, Sigmund Freud. Freud would probably not have separated Kim's suffering into the distinct worlds of thyroid, on the one hand, or psychosis, on the other. For Freud, they would be directly connected.

In chapter 3 I examined the connection between dramatic variations in the inner pulse and blood glucose. Studies have shown that glucose levels can affect personality, and my patient demonstrated the truth that personality can determine glucose levels. With the thyroid gland, the connection between mind and body is not as obvious, and it is not well known in either medical or psychiatric literature the extent to which thyroid function may affect a patient's deep intuition.

The prevailing wisdom is that there is not a direct connection. John was not alone in thinking of these issues as separate. As Robin Hogarth wrote in *Educating Intuition*, "It should be noted of course, that not all changes in the body lead to instinctive behavior. Take the thyroid gland, for example. This secretes an enzyme that regulates, through the bloodstream, many important functions such as the rate at which your heart beats. For different reasons, the thyroid gland may change its level of activity at a given point in a person's life and affect the person's metabolism. (It can become too 'slow' or too 'fast.') However, unlike hunger, changes in the activity of our thyroid gland do not induce thoughts that tell us to do something about it. Indeed, people do not usually even know they have a thyroid problem until they have undergone explicit medical tests. Whereas we do engage in instinctive behavior when the level of our blood sugar drops, we do not possess instinctive reactions to changes in the activity level of our thyroid gland."

I disagree with Hogarth's statement because of the lesson I learned from Kim. Her case was a dramatic example of how a thyroid disruption can alter a patient's intuitive radar, affecting the inner pulse.

Doctors often fail when their usual pattern of diagnostic thinking doesn't solve a problem. The National Institutes of Health has developed the Undiagnosed Diseases Program, in which brilliant NIH investigators led by William Gahl can try their hand at solving medical mysteries. Yet would a real-life Dr. House have solved a problem like Kim's, or would Gahl and his group have joined John and simply pegged her as someone with a psychiatric problem?

Kim's case is an object lesson in how doctors tend to be too rigid when we approach our patients from the vantage point of our particular specialty. I was just beginning to learn to be open-minded enough to close my medical eyes and dance in the dark, letting my patient lead.

The doctor is your guide, but you are in charge, and your inner pulse holds the key. In the end, Kim's preoccupations led me to the truth.

7

Infection of Body, Infection of Spirit

For the strength of the Pack is the Wolf, and
the strength of the Wolf is the Pack.
—Rudyard Kipling

The inner pulse is very powerful, but it is a human manifestation, and it is subject to damage. Many illnesses produce a negative force that wears away at it.

Your pulse may also be affected by the power of suggestion. What can seem like mundane bacteria one day may appear to be transformed the next day into a potent killer. A society's collective inner pulse is worn down through mass hysteria, when people react with fear about a disease that seems to get stronger. Perception can influence response—in the end, bacteria may end up becoming more powerful due to our perceptions of them. Overuse of antibiotics based on fear of disease can promote more drug resistance in germs because the fittest bacteria survive. The mental perception of the power of a "superbug" can probably also have a negative impact on healing. I believe the weakened inner pulse emotes an expectation of illness that hampers the body's immune response as the bacteria spread.

Juan Morales was an easygoing forty-four-year-old construction worker who came to see me in 2006. At first, his medical problem seemed routine. He had recurrent skin infections that were treatable with antibiotics and small surgical incisions. Although it was true that the bacteria that caused his problem (methicillin resistant staph aureus, or MRSA) posed a logistical challenge by being resistant to several commonly used antibiotics, and he was allergic to some of the ones that did work, he could tolerate a few effective antibiotics.

"Whatever you say, Doc," was Juan's favorite response to my latest treatment. "I got no problem."

He had been dealing with the resistant bacteria for some time but never worried about the flesh-consuming potential until the tabloid media coverage began. Morales had developed a rash when he took oral tetracycline, sulfa drugs, and Zyvox, a newer antibiotic designed specifically to treat this bacteria. He had to be hospitalized twice in the summer of 2007, where he received the gold-standard treatment: the intravenous antibiotic Vancomycin, along with the surgical incision and drainage of an abscess on his buttocks and the soft tissue of his knee. He was completely cured both times.

In the fall of 2007, the media spotlight suddenly shifted to MRSA, and it was renamed a superbug. This created a cloud of fear that obscured the real risk, which was still fairly small. The superbug was only the latest in a series of health scares, although, in Juan's case, the new name alone was enough to change his life and his feelings about himself.

The brushfire of worry about MRSA ignited when a simple fact was reported in the news media and blown out of proportion.

The Centers for Disease Control published a report in October 2007 documenting 94,000 cases of serious MRSA infection, with 19,000 deaths in 2005. Although MRSA had been common in hospitals for decades, the CDC was finally tracking the actual number of infections, which made for the breaking news—and news had to feel new to be convincing. So despite the fact that 85 percent of these infections occurred in hospitals where MRSA had been known for years as a colonizer, rather than the super-bug, and the vast majority of MRSA-threatened patients were already sick or their immune systems already compromised from other diseases, nevertheless we focused on the community infec-tions (15 percent), which suddenly seemed to be rampant and uncontrollable.

Many people were soon afraid to go to their schools and gyms. Fear of the superbug was testament to the media's ability to spin a story until the public felt as if a biblical-type scourge had invaded every community. Reacting to the extensive reporting, people exaggerated and personalized the risk. Small skin infec-tions suddenly loomed as potential death sentences, and lost in all of the sudden concern was the important fact that almost all MRSA cases were treatable.

Morales grew frightened. "I don't want to die, Doc," he said to me on several occasions.

Once the public panic attack started, the list of antibiotics that effectively treated MRSA began to escape media attention. Back in the sober days before the birth of the superbug, when ordinary MRSA was making its way around hospital wards and into gyms and schools, the list of treatments was well known to all practicing infectious disease specialists.

Morales felt as if his life were collapsing. He read, on the front page of the New York Post, about a twelve-year-old Brooklyn boy who died of MRSA. When Morales saw me in late October

2007 for a small skin infection on his leg, he kept nervously looking at the door of my office as if he expected officials from the
state health department to follow him in.

"I have the same bacteria that people are dying from," he said
in an uncharacteristically high-pitched voice. He sat on my examination table fully dressed with his arms folded and his forehead
furrowed. Normally, he didn't need prompting to change into a
patient gown, but now I had to ask him repeatedly to remove his
pants.

The red spot on his leg was only the size of a half dollar,
but he didn't seem reassured when I said that one of the usual
antibiotics would handle it. "There's nothing I haven't told you,"
I said calmly. "This is not a new form of bacteria. Nothing has
changed."

"I don't want to die," he said with panic in his voice.

Everything except the bacteria had changed. Morales now
saw himself as a leper. I found myself washing my hands several
times after seeing him, and I immediately donned my gloves
whenever I was in the same room with him. It was the power of
perception on all sides.

"He has it?" my office manager Jasmine said, and she, too,
looked worried, wiping the exam table and the doorknobs with
alcohol after Morales used them. This was something she didn't
do even for our sickest patients.

I encouraged Morales to see Dr. Roger Dennis, an infectious
disease specialist, and Jasmine arranged an appointment for the
same day. Dennis had a larger quiver of antibiotic arrows that he
could use for this tricky bacteria.

Dennis, an experiential expert who was immune to the fear of
the superbug, called me after he saw Morales and spoke to me in
a calm voice. He prescribed clindamycin, a powerful old-school
antibiotic that sometimes caused gastrointestinal side effects.

Morales responded to the antibiotic, although it seemed to take longer than usual, as if the fear and the stress had weakened his inner pulse. The sinister-seeming bacteria spread to his buttock, and the infection needed to be lanced surgically before it began to heal.

MRSA certainly seemed more potent and powerful these days.

Out on the streets, Juan's friends avoided him as if he had the plague. He told many people about his skin infections, and now he was unable to land any new construction jobs, a librarian told him to go to another library, and both a gas station attendant and a supermarket manager told him to take his business elsewhere.

Morales's girlfriend called me, worried, to ask whether it was risky if they had sex. "No," I reassured her. MRSA is transmissible on the skin, but although Morales's girlfriend had repeatedly been exposed, she hadn't gotten sick. MRSA is a colonizer that often doesn't cause an infection.

As happens with all media-stoked hype, the irrational worry around the superbug gradually abated, and in 2008 and 2009 Morales found himself slowly returning to a calmer world. MRSA no longer seemed as mysterious, and it was clearly not swooping in to decimate the lives of healthy people the way the news reports originally seemed to suggest.

Morales was more relaxed and healthier, and his inner pulse once again signaled health, rather than sickness. His skin infections came less frequently by 2009 and seemed again to be easier to treat. Morales was cured both before and after the public storm, but during the storm, the psychological cost of the cure was far greater.

Fear fills the headlines but is not an effective tool for long-term learning. Fear of bacteria causes an excessive use of antibiotics, which leads to a vicious Darwinian circle: bacteria that mutate and become resistant to antibiotics thrive in an environment of drug overuse.

To battle a resistant bug such as MRSA, first we need to improve the infectious-disease precautions at hospitals. Attention must be given to more hand washing, greater care with sterile equipment, and cleaner rooms and beds. Second, we need to douse the media-stoked flames of fear whenever news hype affects perception the way it did in late 2007 for MRSA. Third, it is important to promote the development of newer antibiotics to treat emerging and resistant bacterial strains that occur.

The true science of superbugs has to be painstaking to be effective. Unfortunately, this is often not the case. The 2007 scare occurred partly because bacteria were allowed to thrive and propagate in hospitals. Boston University researchers who surveyed forty-nine operating rooms at four New England hospitals in 2007 found that cleaners overlooked more than half of the surfaces they were supposed to clean. A much larger study of close to a thousand hospital rooms in Washington, D.C., and New England discovered the same thing. In Texas, a patient became infected with a resistant bug that had lived on an EKG wire for more than a month.

Bacteria can live for almost three months on clothing, an easy vehicle for transmitting them from patient to patient, and a study from the University of Maryland found that the vast majority of doctors change their lab coats less than once a week. This type of neglect is a breeding ground for resistant strains of bacteria. According to a recent report by the FDA, 70 percent of hospital germs had developed resistance to at least one antibiotic.

Recent research suggests that this problem can be improved. When a hospital in Dorchester, England, greatly increased the size of its cleaning staff in 2006, MRSA transmission dropped almost 100 percent during the next six months. A grant from the

Robert Wood Johnson Foundation was used to demonstrate the effectiveness of a social change strategy to both prevent and control the transmission of MRSA. Hospitals in Philadelphia and Pittsburgh, Pennsylvania; Billings, Montana; Baltimore; and Louisville, Kentucky, showed a 23 to 66 percent reduction in MRSA infection rates from 2005 to 2007 with this strategy.

In addition to improved strategies for disinfection and infection containment, new antibiotics are also clearly needed, but most drug companies aren't motivated to develop them.

"Most existing antibiotics are as old as the earth, screened out of nature where they resided, doing battle with bugs for centuries," Dr. Scott Gottlieb, the former deputy commissioner of the FDA, wrote in the *Wall Street Journal* on October 30, 2007. "We need to accelerate this evolution in our laboratories." Unfortunately, there has been an on-again, off-again public response to contagion that has led to far-from-optimal public health. Based on public perception, plans and solutions are too often oversized or undersized, depending on the fears of the moment.

Human beings fear the unknown because it reminds us of the mystery that shrouds the greatest of all of our fears—the fear of our own deaths. New and exotic-sounding diseases scare us deeply, affecting our inner pulse, as we connect these supposed dangers to the sense of our own mortality. A more rational assessment of health risks would involve the likelihood of various scenarios actually happening. Yet most of us are ruled by our emotions and lack perspective on health issues. We perceive risks through the echo chamber of ever-expanding media outlets.

Evidence from several studies supports the notion that emotions affect a person's susceptibility and response to infection. In one study, patients who reported a high level of stress or negative moods got sicker when they were exposed to respiratory viruses than did subjects who were calm or happy. In another study, an association was found between negative emotions and an increased susceptibility to colds.

Ironically, it turns out that excessive worry that viruses or bacteria can make you sick appears to increase the likelihood that they can, because worry interferes with your immune protection against them.

Bacteria are easy targets for worry. They are only a few microns in size, invisible to the naked eye. It is easy to either forget about them entirely or become overly fearful of them, imagining that they are about to attack.

These stressful reactions of suddenly perceived vulnerability made Morales and others more susceptible to infection. The fortitude to resist or not to resist resides in the strength or the weakness of a patient's inner pulse. The MRSA did not actually become more powerful when the media frenzy erupted; it only appeared to gain strength as the inner pulse weakened from worry.

We need to be aware. Stress and negative emotions may wear away at our inner pulse. Keeping our immune systems strong is vital to our well-being.

8

Never Say Die

When your desires are strong enough you
will appear to possess superhuman powers
to achieve.

—Napoleon Hill

As I passed the breast cancer–screening center on First
Avenue in the spring of 2006, I walked behind a small
elderly woman. She seemed familiar, and I wondered whether
it was this familiarity that drew me along. She had a thick mop
of brown hair, her shoulders drooped, and pockets of loose skin
were visible on her neck. Her features were so familiar, I thought
she might be a long-lost relative.

When she made a sudden turn into the cancer-screening center, I realized that she reminded me of my Aunt Vivian, who had
died of lung cancer five years earlier. The similarity was so striking that for a moment, I imagined that she *was* my beloved aunt
who had suffered through a life of lonely nights after her husband
died young of a brain tumor, only to die alone herself of recurrent lung cancer so many years later. I don't believe in ghosts,
but while following this woman, I felt as if I'd briefly reentered

Vivian's life, and I wondered whether this rift in time and space was a signal that I was about to die or become very ill.

It turned out that the woman I followed was a total stranger; as I drew closer, I realized that the similarities between her and my dead aunt were superficial. But soon afterward, as I became heavily involved in the life of my sister's husband's aunt (my sister called her the other Aunt Vivian), I came to see the woman I saw as a premonition of sorts.

Beverly Morel was the aunt of my sister's husband, and like Vivian, she had a honeycomb of thick brown hair and lived as a spinster. My sister had attached herself to Beverly precisely because Beverly reminded her of Vivian, and Beverly often occupied the seat at my holiday dinner table where Vivian had once sat in the years before she died. Beverly was more of an intellectual than Vivian had been, and she craved weekly fixes of music and theater, but, like Vivian, she bore her suffering and loneliness silently and regally, doing her best to punctuate it with social pleasantries and close family ties.

My sister was visiting me from California when Beverly called her to say that she had fainted. I quickly suggested that Beverly go to the emergency room. Her regular internist, who admitted patients to another hospital, wasn't available and hadn't seen her in months.

In the ER, I determined that Beverly had a bad urinary tract infection that required intravenous antibiotics. She had probably blacked out because of dehydration. Unfortunately, when she fainted she had broken her ankle, which would require surgery, and afterward she would be unable to walk for at least six weeks.

Beverly stayed in the hospital for a month until her insurance coverage ran out. She still couldn't walk or take care of herself after the operation, so I transferred her at her request to Terence

Cardinal Cook, a rehabilitation facility/nursing home. There she developed another urinary tract infection and was started on more antibiotics, which caused her colon to become inflamed. The nursing home doctor didn't diagnose the colon infection right away, and by the time this semi-retired practitioner alerted me to the problem and asked that Beverly be transferred back to the hospital she was already quite ill. By the time she arrived she was already in a coma, her colon was five times its normal size, and she had a white blood cell count that was ten times normal.

The gastroenterologist I consulted, Dr. Jerry Davis, said that he had never seen a colon this bad, and he was positive that the entire organ would have to be removed surgically for her to have any chance to survive. "It's a leaky bag of bacteria," he said. "It will never heal."

Dr. Howard McCormack, the surgeon I called, refused to operate, insisting that the operation itself would open up non-healing tracks of infection known as fistulas and kill her just as quickly. He added that he still believed there was a chance she could improve from medical treatment alone. He was the only doctor on the case who believed it. There was no science, no text-book to back him up on his opinion, just a feeling. McCormack looked into the eyes of his patient, and, somewhat uncharacter-istically for a surgeon, he sensed the inner pulse of a survivor, although he didn't call it that.

Beverly's brother, Tom Morel, was an opinionated research scientist who appointed himself as Beverly's family spokesper-son. He was also her health-care proxy, and he was soon involved with every aspect of the case. He insisted that his sister would never want to live with a colostomy bag and was glad the surgeon wouldn't operate. "She already complains that her life is shit," he said, "without our giving her a bag of it to change every day." Tom returned to his home in western Massachusetts, and left his wife,

Libby, to look after his sister. Libby was less confrontational and easier to deal with. She spent hours at Beverly's bedside every day, whispering into Beverly's ear and keeping her up-to-date on her condition. There was no sign that Beverly heard any of this or responded to it in any way, but I believe it helped Beverly cling to life, much as Gould's sister had helped him cling to life (as I described in chapter 2).

Every day on my rounds I stared into Beverly's vacant eyes and wondered what she would have decided for herself if she were awake. Would she have risked the surgery? I realized that I might never know Beverly's thoughts, because her infection worsened despite the most powerful antibiotics we could offer her. The only effective way to manage such a case was day to day. Changes in the inner pulse, for better or worse, were imperceptible. It was easy to grow impatient, trying to will my patient to recover. Yet daily medicine is like a slow military march across the countryside—it is accomplished step by step. Every morning and every evening, I reviewed Beverly's elevated white blood counts, her bloody diarrhea, her lack of response to my voice or touch, and her persistently elevated temperatures, and I resigned myself to play out the string. Each day another specialist ceased writing notes or coming by to see her, additional signs that doctors did not expect Beverly to survive.

And yet, as she continued to simply lie there, after a while—like the surgeon—I began to develop a growing unscientific intuition that somehow she *was* going to survive. At first, this wasn't supported by any numbers—they had stopped worsening, but they still weren't improving. I wondered irrationally whether Libby and the professionals who were caring for Beverly were somehow willing her back to consciousness. I wasn't alone in my emotional response; every nurse and nurse's aide on Beverly's case was so used to patients like her being killed by pneumonia or gastric bleeds or strokes that they slowly began to root her on. She had so little reserve at this point that almost anything wrong that happened could take her life.

Yet she continued to live. After several days of her surviving against the odds, we all began to believe that she was somehow intended to recover. She was tougher than I'd realized, hanging onto life, gaining little bits of momentum. I began to wonder whether it could be hope, hers and ours, that fueled her inner pulse and kept her going. Hope is an emotion that I believe can have an impact on both neurochemistry and the outcome of a disease.

Beverly had never been a particularly hopeful or religious person, and I didn't think she would have believed that faith could heal her. Talmudic scholars have said that a person over the age of fifty is kept alive by the mitzvahs, or good deeds, that he or she does, and without these, you are basically running on smoke. Before fifty, your youth and a good set of working bodily organs keep you going; after fifty, as you come to be inscribed in the Book of Life every year on Rosh Hashanah, you have to earn your way forward with good deeds. Mitzvahs are food for the inner pulse.

Yet it was hard to picture Beverly in these terms, especially given her predilection for disputes and dislikes; few people pleased her and few situations made her feel comfortable. She was frequently judgmental, often losing friends over petty issues, such as who paid for dinner or who had phoned the other last. Once you had offended her, she had a long memory for it. She was a collector of injustices.

My Aunt Vivian was kinder than Beverly, and when Vivian was granted a six-year reprieve from lung cancer, I always believed that she was being rewarded for her kind heart. In this way Beverly was not like Vivian, who suffered for perfect strangers. Random rapes and shootings hurt Vivian, as if there was supposed to be a true system of justice that applied to everyone, not only to people she knew. After six years, however, lung cancer returned to rapidly reclaim Aunt Vivian's life, whereas Beverly had now persisted for many days in the ICU. Why? Was it somehow predestined for Vivian to die and for Beverly to survive, or did Beverly have a stronger inner pulse?

Calvinists believe that all of life is predestined, that some souls are destined for salvation and others for damnation. Regarding Beverly's story, a Calvinist would say that her unexpected survival had nothing to do with her mental, physical, emotional, or spiritual power; her survival had already been set.

The Roman Catholic view, by contrast, teaches that God wills the salvation of all souls, but certain of us are granted special grace. So Beverly's recovery could be a reward in life for a special deed. Jewish theologians have attempted to reconcile free will with the seemingly contradictory notion that God is all-knowing and all-seeing and is present in the past and the future at the same time. Moses Maimonides explained this apparent contradiction by pointing out that God's knowledge is incorrectly understood as a super version of human knowledge. If a human being were to know beforehand how a man will behave and know it beyond all doubt, that man would not be free to do otherwise. Yet God exists beyond this plan and in his incomprehensible omniscience allows us our free will to make choices, while at the same time knowing and allowing the choices we will make.

Maimonides also believed in a personal God who performs miracles and judges us and rewards us on a moment-to-moment basis. What had Beverly done to be inscribed in the Book of Life, rather than in the Book of Death? The answer was unknowable, although it manifested in her inner pulse and its code for survival, rather than for death.

Looking at Beverly, I found it impossible to know exactly what spiritual or mystical factors had channeled through her inner pulse to keep her heart ticking and her brain transmitting, even when it seemed medically impossible for this to be happening.

Dr. Davis said, "I've never seen a patient survive where a colon is five times normal size and a white blood count is so high. Her colon is a balloon of pus and bacteria. Even if it shrinks, it will leak. Regular food will punch holes in it." Davis was so committed to the view that surgery was Beverly's only chance at survival that even when he saw Beverly's colon start to shrink, her stool become more formed, and her fevers begin to abate, he continued to push the surgeon to operate.

McCormack and Tom Morel, however, remained vocal in their refusals. It was as if all of us, except Davis, could smell a fresher scent in Beverly's room: the scent of recovery. Still asleep, in a lighter coma, moving her arms and legs and beginning to look around the room when her name was yelled, Beverly was finally moved out of intensive care to a bed in the Special Care Unit, a four-bed ward where the nurses were still vigilant. Day by day, Beverly's recovery continued against all odds. Six weeks after her initial transfer back to my hospital from Cardinal Cooke, her white blood count returned to the normal range of under 10,000, and her stool took on real shapes. She no longer had a fever, and she opened her eyes and stared across the room. Her brother, consumed with worry that we would still whisk her off to surgery against her will, came to town to visit and immediately asked a psychiatrist to see her to confirm that she was still incompetent. The psychiatrist, Dr. Goldberg, a veteran of too many hospital wars with irrational families and the same doctor who had previously seen Brian Solomon, now wondered aloud why he was being called to see a patient who was so obviously still delirious.

"The brother thinks there's a conspiracy forcing her to go to surgery," I said.

"Maybe he should see me," said Goldberg.

As it began to look more and more like Beverly might be the one-in-a-million patient to survive this kind of ordeal, I continued to ask myself why. The odds were overwhelmingly against her survival, especially without surgery—yet she continued on. Neither science nor religion could give me a tangible explanation as to *why*. It all came down to the surprising force of her inner pulse, unseen and unmeasurable, but beating ever on. I suddenly realized there was another aspect to Beverly that may have partly explained her recovery. My sister told me that she was stubborn. She didn't like to give up. This wasn't the toughness of a warrior or the thick hide of a politician, but on a day-to day basis perhaps this was what she needed to fight off a severe illness.

The grit of the strong inner pulse kept beating on stubbornly when others predicted that it was supposed to stop. In the end, what Beverly's survival came down to was the accumulation of monotonous, monitor-blipping, infusion-bloating, gray near-death days that, taken together, added up to her recovery.

When she finally opened her eyes and looked around with some recognition of being in the world, I began to ask her questions. Most of my questions had no immediate answers. She still didn't know where she was or the date, and her concerned brother secretly rushed another psychiatrist up to see her to make sure she was still documented as incompetent and that Davis and I weren't trying to pull an end-run around him to push her into surgery.

Beverly continued to live, but her case remained a scientific mystery. By early 2007, she had improved to the point where she was discharged from the hospital and began coming to see me in my office. I felt an urge to ask her then if she knew why she might have been chosen to survive when so many others in her condition had died. I remember that she was sitting on my hard-cushioned examination table, leaning forward, her neck drooping forward without support. She looked uncomfortable, as so many did, exposed to a doctor's whims, clad only in a flimsy cloth examination gown that opened from the back. Still, Beverly seemed much happier than when she had been in the hospital. I wondered whether she knew just how lucky she was to be alive and how close she had been to death. "Do you remember fighting, not wanting to give up?" I asked her.

"I don't have very clear memories of that time," she said. "I know I was very sick."

"You overcame great odds. The gastroenterologist said no one ever recovers from such a severe bowel infection without surgery, and the surgeon said almost no one ever recovers from the surgery. You were boxed in, with no good options."

Beverly looked at me closely but didn't say anything. Her hair was back to its former Eastern European fluffiness—in the hospital, it had been a mat of sweaty straw for months. In the spirit of her recovery, she had had it dyed auburn brown. Her legs were the most obvious reminder of her recent illness: they were still chalk white and swollen to three times their normal size, engorged with fluid seeping from her veins. Critical illness invariably made the veins as flimsy as tissue paper. Beverly stared at me, and I could see that her intelligence and understanding were returning. She no longer resembled the bloated, uncomprehending patient in the ICU. "I don't know what happened," she said. "I don't believe in ghosts, but I have always felt that my dead mother watches over me."

"Maybe she said something to the boss on your behalf," I said, and Beverly nodded. There is a Jewish teaching that says that when a woman's soul rises after death, she may be in a position to bring entreaties to God on a survivor's behalf if she has lived a just life. If the entreaty is successful, God then fuels the inner pulse for further life.

Beverly wasn't sure. "I don't know if it was Mom," she said.

I asked my neighbor Dr. Leon Pachter, the chief of surgery at my hospital, what he thought was the best explanation for Beverly's miraculous recovery. He knew her case well from surgical rounds with McCormack. Leon was an observant Jew, but he didn't automatically see Beverly's miraculous recovery in religious terms, beyond the simple observation that all matters of life and death are ultimately in God's hands. Speaking with Dr. Pachter in the hallway between our apartments, I remarked that McCormack had been right, against all odds.

"No great wisdom. He was just lucky," the chief surgeon said. Pachter was a tall man in his early sixties who maintained his youthful vigor and wrote powerful, passionate essays on Jewish philosophy. It was odd to hear him interpreting an outcome as being due to luck.

Months later, Beverly had become one of my most unpleasant patients. During multiple visits to my office, she always found something to blame me for. Either "Why can't I reach you on your cell phone right away?" or "Why must my legs always be so swollen?" or "I feel like I'm always going to fall."

"You must elevate your legs at night and use your walker during the day," I insisted, but Beverly smiled past me, a tiny frozen smile that was quickly replaced by the next complaint. As the real Beverly resurfaced, it was becoming clear just how self-centered she was. Perhaps *this* was her best survival trait.

In the winter of 2007, Beverly made an unanticipated return to the hospital. While out with friends, she had ignored everyone's advice about walking carefully and had left her cane home. Feeling her new freedom, she went into a Dunkin' Donuts to get coffee for herself and a friend. Twisting to look at a wall photo at the same time that her hands were occupied with the coffee, she tried to use her hips to push open the door. She toppled and immediately broke the opposite leg from the one that had led to her prolonged hospitalization a year earlier. Beverly's family felt angry about her injury, after all that she'd suffered through to get well, but this time no one flew into town to see her. "It's different this time," her brother, Tom, announced. "She's not in the same trouble."

Once again she healed quickly, sitting in her hospital bed with her hands folded and her chin thrust forward, saying, "I'm angry. I'm annoyed about several things." It again occurred to me that it was her pushy, cranky will that powered her inner pulse and kept her going. As I left the room, she was muttering about a lazy nurse's aide and a problem with the food service. It was a revelation for me to consider that the inner pulse—which led to a positive or a negative outcome—could be a dark power, as well as a heavenly one. Libby came to visit from upstate New York for a cameo appearance, and then back to a nursing home Beverly went—the same type of place where the infected bowel had occurred. This time I wasn't worried. Beverly was medical rubber; I knew she would bounce back, no matter what.

Health care is often the world of the unexpected. All of the patients who had come before Beverly and had not recovered from colonic infections as severe as hers led to the textbook way of predicting—wrongly—the outcome of her condition. Parameters that were adhered to by as knowledgeable and experienced a physician as Dr. Davis were based on reading, combined with clinical practice.

When Beverly Morel broke the mold with her unanticipated and uncanny improvement, it stimulated a different kind of medical search into uncharted territory—there was no textbook to read, no physician to consult. There was a search to conduct, but it was a lonely search without another case for corroboration. The question of why Beverly had survived when no one else had eventually led me to examine her particular traits: stubbornness, even obnoxiousness, as well as her own will to live.

Had Libby reached in to stimulate this unseen force to recovery? Had Beverly's dead mother's presence somehow done so? "Don't put too much about my mother in your book," Beverly later warned me, not wanting to jinx this presence by calling too much attention to it.

The main lesson, however, wasn't about the power of ghosts or even the power of will; it was about the power that a patient had as an individual, the power that each of us has to use the force of our will to defy expectations and statistics. Our inner pulse can save us, just as it can kill us.

After Beverly's unexpected recovery, I found myself searching for traits in other patients that might predict their survival from life-threatening illnesses.

What caused one patient to live on after a cancerous brain tumor was removed, while another died almost immediately? The force emanated from the inner pulse, either positive or negative. In the much more common negative case, even after a top brain surgeon might remove a tumor whole and slice out the cancer down to the last visible millimeter, unfortunately, microscopic tentacles of tumor still infiltrated the jellolike tissue of the brain.

James Coyne, PhD, the director of the Behavioral Oncology Program at the Abramson Cancer Center at the University of Pennsylvania School of Medicine, analyzed data using a quality-of-life questionnaire in two studies with more than 1,000 patients who had head and neck cancer. Of the 646 who died, he did not find a difference in survival rate between those who died with or without a positive outlook. "The hope that we can fight cancer by influencing emotional states appears to have been misplaced,"

Coyne told me. Coyne acknowledged that the impact of negative emotion in cardiovascular health had been demonstrated, but not so for cancer. "We don't believe that the tumors grow because we get more upset. If it's the case, there certainly hasn't been any evidence of it. There is also no evidence that psychotherapy, for example, promotes the survival of cancer patients."

Studies have shown that 25 percent of patients with terminal cancer are depressed and that there is a significant improvement in the depression with antidepressant therapy. Yet David Spiegel of Stanford was unable to show that support-expressive group therapy with breast cancer patients improved either psychological distress or outcome. "The bottom line," Coyne said, "is that emotional well-being does not appear to improve cancer survival."

Harvard's Dr. Jerome Groopman, myself, and many other experts would disagree. In his book *The Anatomy of Hope*, Groopman considered the idea that positive emotions like hope can lead to a better immune response and perhaps better tumor fighting in some patients. Conversely, negative emotions may impair a patient's ability to fight cancer.

Why do some people live when so many others die of a horrible condition? And is there a way to tell the difference?

After many years in practice, I was finally developing the ability to look at a patient and quickly assess his or her vitality—to gauge his or her spiritual essence and whether it was waxing and waning. This was a quick take on the inner pulse, and it seemed to have some value in predicting healing.

I asked Dr. Michael Gruber, a neuro-oncologist, a specialist in brain cancer, whether he could tell the difference between the many who had died of terminal brain cancer and the few who lived. I encountered him in the garage of my apartment building where we both parked our cars. It was a crisp spring day in

April 2008. He was wearing his usual immaculately pressed suit and designer glasses, and his wavy hair was well combed.

Looking at him, I found it difficult to guess that he gave chemotherapy to patients with malignant brain tumors who were generally dead in fewer than two years. "Have you ever had someone with a glioblastoma live?" I asked.

"I have seventeen patients," he said, "who have survived with incurable brain cancer for ten years already."

"How?"

"We don't know. All had their tumors resected, and all received radiation. All had chemo, most of it the stuff that never works. Yet all are doing okay, without recurrence."

Gruber was treating one of my patients, Smiling Sy Jones, a famous reggae music agent. So far, he was one of the lucky ones.

"Your patient's doing well," he said. "A year so far. He could be number eighteen."

"Is there anything the group has in common? Are they stronger physically? Do they all have the same positive attitude about life that Sy has?" I pressed.

Gruber sighed, revealing the mental weight of his chosen field. "I don't know. They seem to share a will to live," he said. "Most are positive and say they are going to beat their tumor. A few have survived on the experimental drugs [Thalidomide and Temodar]. Even the best brain surgeons can't get it all. But there is something about the immune system of the survivors that gets them through it."

Dr. Gruber was giving the new cancer drug Avastin to patients with promising results, and he was also testing a revolutionary technique known as an autologous vaccine: a portion of the patient's tumor was used to make antibodies against itself. This vaccine was unique for each patient. A patient would be treated for more than three years with the vaccine, as well as with growth factors. It had been studied in twelve patients so far. "It's too early to know," he said. "But 26 percent have survived for two years, a tremendous improvement."

Beyond the will to live and a strong immune system, what did patients who survived against long odds have in common? Gruber hesitated. "Sometimes I think all surviving patients are tough. Sometimes I think they're all just very positive. Sometimes I think you have to be obnoxious as hell to fight off this kind of cancer. And sometimes I think it's all luck."

Maybe sometimes it's the patient's spirit that just refuses to die.

9

Radar to Live

What medicines do not heal, the lance will;
what the lance does not heal, fire will.

—*Hippocrates*

The inner pulse is the most powerful force in the body, connected to a greater spiritual reality, a window simultaneously into the body and the soul, but, as I've shown, it is difficult to define. It can be described but not measured, it is connected directly to intuition and instinct, and it informs a patient, as well as his or her receptive healer.

The inner pulse links each story of this book, although the manifestations are different in each case. Sometimes sensing a patient's inner pulse can be a path to discovering a life-threatening condition. If the condition isn't found in time, death occurs. If it is found, there may be a chance of a cure. Sensing the pulse is of value to a patient.

Many people are led to religious faith. If a person can make peace with God, an inner peace is achieved; the inner pulse resonates with this spiritual truth. This equanimity may be valuable in facing the specter of death. Both Christianity and Judaism have taught that instead of fearing death, we should fear God. A central passage in Jewish teaching states *"Raisheet chochmah yirat Adonoy"* or "The beginning of wisdom is the awe of God."

When Jeremy Kahn first came to see me in early 2001, he immediately said he knew something was wrong with his chest. He was worried and sleepless. He didn't complain of coughing or any problems with breathing. I could find nothing wrong with his physical examination, his lab test results, or his chest X-ray. Science would say that he was fine and didn't require further testing. Yet because he was a smoker, I followed his lead and decided to order a screening CT scan of the lungs just to make certain that there wasn't a hidden problem. Small lung cancers are often too small to be seen on a chest X-ray. The use of screening CT scans of the lungs in smokers has long been controversial, though in 2010, a large National Cancer Institute study showed a significant survival advantage in patients who were screened.

Back in 2001, I didn't have a bad feeling when I ordered the test, but Kahn did.

His intuitive radar (emanating from the inner pulse) was on target. The CT scan showed a tiny lesion at the top of his lung, and a needle biopsy confirmed that it was cancerous. He had an operation to remove the cancer, which went well.

About a month later, I received a phone call on Saturday evening, just past dusk. Kahn had decided to call me right after the conclusion of the Sabbath. His voice was still a hoarse whisper from the effects of the breathing tube that had been stuck down his throat during and after surgery, and I didn't recognize him at first.

"Thank you, Doctor," he whispered. "I know lung cancer can kill you, but you found it very early. Stage IA. No lymph nodes. No spread. I'm clean. A few weeks of chemo, and hopefully I'm done. Thank God."

I recalled the moment when Kahn's appreciation at the early diagnosis had given way to complaints about the disorganization at my hospital. He was kept waiting on a cold chair for more than an hour, and the needle biopsy had to be repeated three times to confirm the suspected result. As a result of these difficulties, he had decided to have his surgery at the somewhat more presti-gious Memorial Sloan-Kettering Cancer Center. I hadn't expected to hear from him again after that. "It's a good thing you came in when you did," I said now, "and we ordered the CT scan. How are you feeling?"

"I'm weak. Very weak. But I'm also very grateful, Doctor."

From a medical perspective, I felt good about the diagnosis and the treatment plan, although not all doctors agreed that smokers such as Kahn should have their lungs screened with CT scans. I knew they were wrong. If I had not screened Kahn, his aggressive cancer would almost certainly have spread beyond the lung. Then he would have been facing metastases to the liver—which might have been barely operable—or to the bone or the brain, which wouldn't have been curable by surgery. Either way, even if he continued to live just as long with the cancer, he would almost certainly have been wracked with pain and chained to debilitating, expensive treatments. By contrast, his current life held the hope of a complete cure.

Two weeks after his phone call to me, he returned to my office, covered with perspiration and breathing shallowly. His hair seemed grayer, and his tiny eyeglasses were crooked and greasy. A quick physical showed me that all of his vital signs were stable, his lungs were clear, and he had a normal temperature.

As he was lounging on my blue office couch, seeming to be in too much pain to sit straight up, he admitted to me the purpose of his visit. He was still under the direct care of the Sloan-Kettering surgeon, but he was coming back to me as a kind of medical good luck charm: I was the one who had made the timely diagnosis. I was familiar with this response—families came if a member was cured while under my care; they left me if someone died.

Yet Kahn also had a deeply spiritual reason for returning.

"I would like to tell you something, Doctor," he said, ready to confide a secret. "I see you as a man of science, not mysticism." His heavily accented voice added intrigue to the statement.

"I hope I am open-minded," I said.

"You know I am observant, a regular congregant at my synagogue. But what you don't know is about my deep interest in the oral tradition of the Jews, the Kabbalah. Have you heard of the mystical rabbis?"

Kabbalah, in Hebrew, means "to receive." It refers to the verbal communication between God and Moses that spawned mystical interpretations of scripture between the seventh and the eighteenth centuries. "Yes, the Kabbalists," I said.

He smiled and continued, "Twelve years ago, Rachamim [the name means "mercy"], a Kabbalist rabbi as you call him, told me that I was supposed to die, but that God was going to have compassion on me and spare me. I've always remembered that, although I wasn't sure how much I believed it at the time.

"But now this year . . . It was two weeks before Rosh Hashanah, two weeks before I was to be inscribed in the Book of Life for the year and my fate determined by God, a week before you ordered the fateful CT scan, 'as a precaution,' you said, and I remember I had a big fight with my wife. We came home from synagogue on Shabbat, and she said we had no life except the shul. We argued about it, and she was very upset, and I went out again, but I had nowhere else to go, so I returned to the synagogue. It was the end of Shabbat, and I saw that there was a mystical rabbi there, a famous rabbi from Israel, and there was a long line of people waiting to speak to him, waiting to hear what he had to say. I stood at the end of the line, and by the time the rabbi got to me I could see through the windows that it was very dark outside. Shabbat was over. When he saw me, I could tell that he was taken aback. I was nervous seeing a sage rabbi looking shaken. He told me that he was going to give me a new name, Mordecai."

"Why a new name?" I asked.

Kahn smiled. "It's a tradition. It signifies a new life. He was telling me that I required a new identity. He said that sometimes things don't go right in life, and God may give you the opportunity to start a new one. He said that he would write me a blessing on parchment and mail it to me from Israel."

"What happened?"

"When I got the results of the CT scan from you, I knew that this was what he had meant. That he had a deep vision or intuition about my cancer. That he looked inside me and saw it. My wife said it was superstition, that these rabbis were just unreliable fortune-tellers, but I didn't agree. I telephoned the rabbi in Israel. I asked if he remembered me, and he said he did. I asked him what he saw, why he gave me another name. He said, 'In reincarnation, sometimes you come into this world with a sentence, something that hangs over your head from a previous life. But God gives you the means to undo that sentence, a medicine to treat it with. Your life has been spared. God will have compassion on you, and there will be a new life for you, and you will be okay.'

I told him the results of the CT scan, and he said again that he could see into my future, and I would be okay. Strangely, the day of the operation, his letter arrived with the parchment and the blessing."

I had contributed to Kahn's well-being by discovering his cancer. Another doctor had swiftly removed the cancer with his scalpel and brought the real chance for a cure. Medical science had found his cancer and cured it, yet in the end, Kahn was most comforted by the notion that both his illness and his recovery had been predicted by the prescient powers of the mystical rabbis. Seen from this perspective, the inner pulse is a transcendent religious power, a direct connection to God. The mystical rabbi could see it better than any doctor could. Giving over control to the rabbi's far-seeing vision had helped Kahn cope and make the difficult transition from apparent health to life-threatening illness and back again in a short period of time.

In the wake of his diagnosis and successful treatment, what gave Kahn the most relief from his growing fear of cancer recurrence was not the statistic that 60 percent of large cell cancers found at this early stage were curable by surgery. Rather, he felt most reassured by the miraculous vision of the mystic.

Yet despite his faith, he still had pangs of worry. He felt fatigued—was this the cancer coming back? Follow-up CT scans showed no recurrence.

Kahn returned to work, then left again, battling depression. Antidepressants helped temporarily, but then he decided to move his entire family, his wife and his three boys, to Israel.

He returned to the United States for medical check-ups, the first in early August 2002. That week the Haftorah, readings from the prophets, was Eikele, a powerful passage of consolation from the prophet Isaiah. Eikele presents God's message of solace and hope to the Children of Israel during the dark times following the loss of the Temple. The portion begins, "But Zion said, the Lord hath forsaken me, and the Lord hath forgotten me." To this, God responds and informs the Jewish people that they are gravely mistaken. God says, "Can a mother ever forget her child; cease to have compassion for him? Even if she could, I will never forget you."

Kahn drew hope and sustenance from this prophecy, and it improved his spirits. God would not forsake him. His religious beliefs grew stronger, and I believed that his inner pulse was bounding.

Kahn's inner pulse had prompted the strong intuition that caused him to seek medical attention in time for an early diagnosis, and this same pulse fueled the faith that helped him to survive the anxiety-fraught years that followed.

Five years after his diagnosis, Kahn continued to fly to New York from Israel every year. Five years without cancer recurrence made him feel calmer, and he talked about opening a small business in Tel Aviv. He was getting along well with his wife, and on his most recent visit, he happily asked me for a prescription for Viagra.

He still spoke of the prescient wisdom of the mystical rabbis. His treatment had combined equal ingredients of fear, intuition, science, and religion. The mixing bowl for this potent brew was his inner pulse.

Richard Sloan, a professor of behavioral medicine at Columbia and the author of *Blind Faith*, told me that Kahn's story of faith and a cure obeyed an essential separation between church and medicine. Both science and mysticism played essential roles, but they were not in competition, and emotions and revelations were not confused with the need for curative surgery.

Sloan was concerned about what in *Blind Faith* he called "the brave new world of religion and health, where science, medicine, faith and ethics exist together in a potentially explosive mixture." Sloan pointed out in his book that faith healing has generally not been shown to work independently of the latest science; he was concerned when faith healing interferes with the sanctity of the doctor-patient relationship. In Kahn's case, this would be the equivalent of the mystical rabbi calling me on the phone and trying to influence the course of Kahn's treatment based on prophecy. Yet at the same time, Sloan acknowledged that the inner pulse, as I termed it, could lead to unexpected cures that defy scientific predictions.

Both Kahn and I stood in awe of the rabbi's wisdom and his vision of the future and found it to be a valuable directive, but we would never seek him out for direct care.

The rabbi was in the tradition of the great Maimonides, who was an inspiration for the integration of the spiritual and the physical. Maimonides was a healer and a Talmudic scholar as well as an early medical scientist. He wrote extensively in all realms, but although his inquiries and discoveries were distinct, nevertheless he was frequently consulted to perform acts of physical healing at his synagogue.

Sloan accepted the idea that a great doctor could also be a visionary rabbi, but he was concerned when religious fervor too easily took the place of a doctor's responsibility to discuss treatment options with his or her patient. As Sloan wrote eloquently, "Because medical patients very often are in pain and fearful, they are especially vulnerable to manipulation by physicians who, even in these days of medical consumerism, retain positions of authority in the physician-patient relationship. When doctors capitalize on this authority to pursue a religious, rather than a medical, agenda, they violate ethical standards of patient care. No one disputes that for a great many people, religion provides comfort in times of difficulty, whether illness-related or otherwise. But being a medical professional means assuming certain responsibilities and foremost among them is acting in the interests of your patients, rather than allowing your personal religious beliefs to interfere."

Nevertheless, it is clear to me, if not to Sloan, that real miracle cures do occur, and that powerful prophets can often see a deadly threat to one's health that a man of science might not be aware of. Mystical insights are important to healing, and they can defy science, even as they provide a connection to the inner pulse.

Only if a cancer is detected before it escapes the lung is there a chance for a surgical cure. Finding this cancer in time is sometimes about a patient's and a doctor's intuition and sensing the inner pulse.

When should I order a CT scan? The answer is different from one patient to the next. A patient's strong emotional response to a perceived threat can be highly useful in first prompting him or her to seek the cause of a life-threatening disease and later to seek the cure. If only the doctor, as William Carlos Williams wrote, is listening.

10

The Black Swan

I believe that in the heart of each human being there is something which I can only describe as a child of darkness who is equal and complementary to the more obvious child of light.

—*Laurens van der Post*

In Thomas Mann's novella *The Black Swan*, Rosalie, a vain woman of fifty, approaches menopause. Battling to retrieve her sexuality and her youth from the inevitability of aging and death, she compares herself to the biblical Sarah, who conceived a child at ninety and laughed at the incongruity (the child was famously called Yitzchak, which in Hebrew means "to laugh"). Rosalie woos a young lover and mistakes the return of her menstrual flow to be a triumph of mind over flesh, as if her anticipated new love has literally restored her physical womanhood. As she rushes to meet him, anticipating their first tryst, she is startled by the appearance of a black swan swimming in the water along her route. She takes some of the stale bread that her young man has brought to feed the bird and eats it herself, which causes the bird to "spread its dark wings and beat the air with them, stretching out its neck and hissing angrily up at her." It soon becomes clear that Rosalie is not experiencing rejuvenation at the hands of her young friend. The return of her period is because her womb is riddled with cancer, and the swan is the Angel of Death.

Rosalie finally acknowledges nature's warnings. Mann wrote, "Pains . . . are usually the danger signals by which nature, always benignant, warns that a disease is developing in the body—look sharp there, it means, something's wrong, do something about it quick, not so much against the pain as against what the pain indicates." Rosalie has missed the warning, and as her period returns for the second time, this time it is as a life-ending hemorrhage.

As Mann's character demonstrates, a woman's menstrual flow can be a sign of life or death, of a healthy womb or a diseased one. A patient can sense a crucial change to her inner pulse and mistake its meaning.

Sylvia Weinstein had been a college student in Buffalo at the same time that I attended SUNY-Buffalo Medical School in the 1980s. We became friends and met occasionally for coffee or a meal. When we both moved to New York, we stayed in e-mail contact.

One day in 1995, Sylvia showed up unannounced at my office and said she wanted to be my patient. She was crying but refused to tell my office manager at the time, Mona, what the problem was. Mona, a well-trained nurse from South America, knew that I was willing to accept my friends as patients.

When I spoke with Sylvia in the waiting room, she told me that she'd suddenly felt weak and dizzy while passing the sign for my office. She didn't look so weak that she might collapse on the spot, but under the bright light of my examination room, I took a closer look. Although she was thirty-five, Sylvia still appeared to be in her late twenties. She was an artist, and her blue denim shirt and khaki pants were stained with red and yellow blotches.

Her long hair was also speckled with paint. She declined to put on one of my blue-cloth patient gowns. She sat far forward on the examining table, moving her feet back against the metal and biting her lower lip.

When I asked her what the problem was, she said that she had been feeling fatigued and stressed. I discovered that she had experienced irregular menstrual periods for most of the previous year. She said that she often missed her period altogether; at other times, it came either early or late. During some months, she even had an extra period. I said that it was possible that her menstrual problems were related to her symptoms of dizziness and fatigue.

Zeroing in on the physical symptoms without considering the precipitating stressors can be a mistake because the mind is so powerful. Thomas Mann's Rosalie had the opposite problem, obsessing on the power of the mind and missing the fact that it was her body that was betraying her. The inner pulse is the fulcrum, the place where mind and body meet and health or disease is determined. It was too early to know what the overriding dynamic was in Sylvia's case.

As she grew more accustomed to our new relationship with me as her doctor, she seemed less embarrassed or shy about her problems. She said she believed that the stress of being an artist was causing the menstrual irregularities. Things always got worse, she explained, just before her paintings were due to appear in a gallery. I knew that hormones can be very sensitive to stress.

By the mid-1990s, I was learning to pay more attention to my patients' instincts and their grasp of their own inner pulses. The hormones that regulate the menstrual cycle, estrogen and progesterone, fluctuate widely and may be directly affected by changes in mood. Conversely, mood may be altered by rapid or extreme fluctuations in the hormones, which can occur when the menstrual cycle is out of whack. I said that I was also concerned that toxins from paint might interfere with her hormone regulation.

"I've never heard that before," she said.

"It hasn't been proven," I told her.

Sylvia's physical examination seemed normal. Her EKG showed no abnormalities, and I told her I would check her blood work to make sure she had no anemia, metabolic abnormalities, or thyroid problems that could also explain her weakness or dizziness. I suggested that she see a gynecologist about her irregular periods as soon as possible.

"Don't you have an answer?" she asked, sounding frustrated.

"I will figure it out," I said. "I will have the lab results back in two days, and you should call me if you start to feel worse."

"But you haven't finished examining me yet," she protested.

I had examined only her heart, lungs, liver, and lymph nodes, perhaps because I still wasn't sure whether she was more of a friend or a patient, but now, with my nurse in attendance, she agreed to put on a gown, and I completed the physical, including an examination of her breasts. I was surprised to find that her breasts were not as fully developed as I'd expected and that her nipples were somewhat recessed, more like the nipples of a man than a woman.

"Have you noticed a change here?" I asked her softly, and she replied that her shrinking breasts disturbed her and her husband the most.

"I want to see the hormone levels," I said.

Two days later, I reviewed the lab results. There was no sign of anemia, dehydration, or metabolic problems. Thyroid hormone levels were normal. The rest of the hormone results would be available the following week. When I called Sylvia with the news, she told me that she had started to see a psychotherapist.

"Do you think it's in my head?" she said.

"No," I said, "I don't. I want to see what the gynecologist says."

Stress might be part of Sylvia's problem, but it wasn't the entire explanation. Her career as a struggling artist was certainly stressful, but at first this didn't seem to be her most overriding health problem. Excess stress hormones, as I discussed in my book *False Alarm*, can lead to a deterioration of the body as well as of the mind. In Sylvia's case, though, I was more concerned about her reproductive hormones. Later that week Sylvia saw her gynecologist, Dr. Sherri Leonard. I called her to discuss Sylvia and suggested that we form a team to take care of her. Leonard had a high-pitched voice and spoke casually, her vocabulary loaded with slang that I was not used to encountering in a physician. I asked her about the changes in Sylvia's breasts, but she said that she wasn't as concerned as I was. "Could be a normal variant," she said. I didn't like this term, especially when a patient wasn't feeling well, and I was afraid that Dr. Leonard's imperiousness could lead her to override a patient's essential intuition.

"What else could it be?" I persisted, and then Leonard admitted that there were several possibilities for Sylvia's irregular menses, including ovarian cysts, uterine polyps, and fibroids. Such growths on the ovary or within the uterus could cause irregular periods. Yet when Leonard performed an ultrasound and a biopsy of the uterine lining, she found no signs of these problems. I told her that I had drawn blood tests for Sylvia's hormone levels and was waiting for the results. Leonard said that she was thinking of starting Sylvia on birth control pills to help make her period "more regular."

A few days later, Sylvia's reproductive hormone levels came back abnormal, which was a shock. At thirty-five, Sylvia seemed to be entering menopause. Estrogen is produced by the ovaries. Sylvia's estrogen level was very low, and her pituitary gland had responded by making more follicle-stimulating hormone (FSH)— trying to flog the ovaries to make more estrogen. Her ovaries were clearly resistant to these hormonal instructions. This scenario was very unusual in a young woman. The normal scenario is that copious amounts of estrogen made by the ovaries signal the brain to turn the FSH meter off.

Sylvia's eggs were not maturing, and estrogen was not being produced. The pituitary kept pumping out more and more FSH to stimulate estrogen to be made, but to no avail, a vicious cycle that was getting her nowhere. It was like a heater that won't turn off in a drafty house because no actual heating is taking place.

Menopause usually occurs in middle age, when the ovaries run out of most of their eggs and cannot produce estrogen, despite high FSH levels telling them to do so. Although a female baby is born with several million eggs, nearly half will have atrophied by the time she reaches puberty. After that, eggs compete every month within each ovary to mature; the winning egg is released into the fallopian tube and the losing eggs atrophy. By the age of forty-five or fifty, a woman has usually exhausted her supply of viable eggs. In cases of premature menopause, some eggs may remain, but they are unable to function or mature.

Perhaps stress was the best explanation. It was possible that stress and fatigue had altered her hormones. Sylvia hadn't yet experienced the full hot flashes—the intermittent rapid dilation of blood vessels—that often ensue as estrogen levels fall during menopause.

I called Dr. Leonard to tell her the news, but she was away on vacation. I spoke with the doctor who was covering her. My secretary Mona faxed the results to Dr. Leonard's office.

Sylvia skipped her follow-up appointment with me, and Mona was unable to reach her by telephone. I hoped that Dr. Leonard was taking care of her problem. I called her and left a message, but she never returned my call.

Three months later, Sylvia suddenly reappeared, again without an appointment, and Mona fit her into my schedule. I was glad to see her, but in the examining room, Sylvia looked very angry.

"Are your periods still irregular?" I asked her.

Tears streamed down Sylvia's face. Apparently, Dr. Leonard had kept her on birth control pills and kept saying that she had nothing to worry about. Sylvia felt intimidated.

"Did she say you might be entering menopause?"

"She mentioned it but said she didn't think it was the most likely explanation."

I didn't tell Sylvia my feeling that Leonard had allowed crucial months to pass without a good treatment plan. "Why didn't you call me back or come to your appointments?"

"I told Dr. Leonard that since we were friends, that maybe it was better if she were the one to treat me. She said that was okay, because the problem was more in her field."

Sylvia said that the birth control pills had worked temporarily, because her cycles became regular for a few months. Now that she had stopped taking the pills, however, her periods had ceased altogether.

In a normal menstrual cycle, surges of estrogen from an ovary help an egg mature and finally break out of its follicle, or small sac, and enter the fallopian tube for the three-day journey to the womb. Two weeks later, the ruptured egg sac produces a surge of the hormone progesterone, which helps prepare the lining of the womb to receive a fertilized egg. This progesterone also suppresses the maturation of an egg in the other ovary.

Today's birth control pills consist largely of progesterone mixed with some estrogen. By taking birth control pills, a woman artificially boosts the level of progesterone during most of her cycle, thus preventing eggs in both ovaries from maturing. If an egg doesn't mature, it doesn't leave the ovary and the woman doesn't ovulate. If she doesn't ovulate, she can't get pregnant.

For the last seven days of the cycle, however, the birth control pills contain no progesterone. This drop-off prompts the uterus to shed its lining, causing the bleeding of menstruation. In Sylvia's case, taking the pills had made her bleed again, but it only seemed as if she was back to normal. She still had the estrogen problem, and without her own estrogen, her eggs were still not capable of maturing.

Sitting on the blue couch in my consultation room, Sylvia told me that her husband was eager to start a family. She had resisted becoming pregnant for the first five years of her marriage in order to pursue her career. Now that her periods had stopped, she realized for the first time just how much she wanted to have children. "It's the first time I've ever looked forward to my period," she said.

I told her that I believed she might be entering menopause early. There was still some chance that premature menopause could be reversed, but Sylvia would have to see a hormone expert.

I referred Sylvia to Dr. Blanche Garber, a fertility and reproductive hormone specialist. Dr. Garber was a kind doctor who was good at presenting a problem honestly but without making the patient feel afflicted. She could preserve hope without exaggerating it. I believed she felt for her patient's inner pulse and connected with it.

Dr. Garber told me that Sylvia probably still had some eggs, but she thought the chances of reversing the menopause were very slight.

Dr. Garber had a plan. She explained to Sylvia that she could begin to take estrogen alone to see whether it would restart the motor and stimulate normal ovarian function, but the chances were very slim. Sometimes periods resumed, with or without estrogen. Much more often, however, they never returned in a woman who was experiencing premature menopause.

Menopause in a woman of thirty-five was rare. Dr. Garber told Sylvia that more women were being diagnosed with this condition than ever before. Perhaps, she said, the problem was occurring more often because more women were delaying child-bearing into their thirties.

What had caused it in Sylvia's case? I called Joan Garber and asked her opinion. Could it be due to stress, coupled with toxins from paint?

"It's a possibility," Dr. Garber said. "That theory has never been proved but I believe it."

When I next saw Sylvia, she had been taking estrogen for two months. She reported feeling calmer, although she still wasn't getting her period. "But my breasts are back," she said, smiling at her own choice of words. She said that her husband had remained supportive.

"I now know that he really loves me," she said.

For the first time in months she seemed well, rather than sick, and if the inner pulse were a real pulse that could be measured, I was sure that hers would be bounding.

Her hair and clothes were no longer streaked with paint. She said that she had been unable to concentrate on her painting. She also said that she now believed that paint toxins might have contributed to her problem, and she needed to figure out a way to minimize them.

Sylvia said she felt more ready than ever to have a child. She told me that she felt cheated by nature, unfairly punished with infertility for having devoted herself to her art. She was also angry with herself for not having decided on motherhood sooner. Now her reproductive engine was stalled. "I feel so helpless," she said. "Time has run out on me."

"Maybe there's still time," I said.

A month later, Sylvia stopped by my office to tell me that her period had resumed, at least for a month. She said she was working closely with Dr. Garber. "She thinks I may be ovulating again," Sylvia added. "She says it's very rare but possible."

A hormone test showed that Sylvia's progesterone levels had risen once at midcycle, a strong sign that Sylvia's ovaries were beginning to function normally again. If the process continued, Dr. Garber would take her off the estrogen and see what happened.

Sylvia said that she was going to try to conceive if she could, and if not, she would adopt an orphan. While smiling over the news, I couldn't help noticing that the streaks of paint had returned to her clothes.

"You're painting again," I said.

Sylvia leaned across the desk, thrusting her shoulders and chin in a way that communicated her determination. She said that she had rented a studio, so she no longer had to work at home. She was also painting with watercolors, rather than oils. Her new paintings were being shown in a major gallery up town. She was going to pursue both children and a career.

"I have to paint," she said. "It's what I do."

It was clear to me that Sylvia had seen herself as sick before. The effects of stress and worry had combined with the toxins to make her ill. As she got better, she began to nurture her inner pulse until it grew stronger. Now that she was well, her inner pulse was providing a buffer around her fragile fertility. The treatment—short-term estrogen, combined with life adjustment—was working. Sylvia's intuition and deep spiritual knowledge of her condition had led her toward an unexpected cure.

David C. Clarke, MD, believes that stress is its own illness. A gastroenterologist who practices medicine in Portland, Oregon, he has studied this phenomenon in more than seven thousand patients and developed a language and a unique approach to the problem, which he says is difficult to measure. Clarke is the author of *They Can't Find Anything Wrong*. He told me in an interview that traditional doctors typically overlook these issues and fall into the rut of asking the same questions again and again, before finally assuming that the symptoms have no basis in medical fact. (Dr. Jerome Groopman brilliantly describes this doctor-with-blinders phenomenon in *How Doctors Think*. Groopman is convinced that the inability of doctors to think outside the box leads to many mistaken diagnoses.)

Clarke has created a larger box for doctors to think in, a whole new set of questions that doctors can and should ask when considering stress as a direct factor in illness. Not all of these questions exist within the confines of traditional science, but they are crucial nevertheless and point toward a greater truth. Stress disorders or stress-related diseases are prominent features in patients' personal and professional lives. Stress has a major effect on both job performance and personal satisfaction. Clarke's goal is to reach the underlying causes of the stress and then to provide a therapeutic milieu for stress relief. Often the stress is due to an abusive or unhappy relationship in the patient's past. This therapeutic milieu counters any suppressed outrage from prior abuses by providing "positive, mutually supportive relationships to replace them."

Clarke has found that physical symptoms may fade if stress is dealt with first, much as I discovered with Sylvia. Patients who feel controlled by their circumstances respond well to what Clarke calls "self-care." In addition to relaxation techniques and exercise, he prescribes at least four hours per week of an activity that makes a patient feel good about himself or herself. These activities range from common relaxation techniques such as prayer, meditation, or yoga to the unusual practice of writing letters to people who you think have abused you.

Many patients under stress know that something is going wrong with their bodies long before any tests or even the best doctor's instincts pick up that there is a problem. Some patients, like Sylvia, are intuitively correct, whereas others, such as Mann's Rosalie, are wrong. Their body radar is broken. As a physician, I must decide whose instincts to trust the most. Over time, I've begun to develop a feel for the appearance of the abnormal and the ability to separate it out from the normal. This medical radar is a crucial part of becoming a healer. It worked for me with James Gould and Kim Bradley, but it wasn't sophisticated enough to help me with Connie Jones's multiple personalities.

There are many practitioners, both doctors and nurses, who have better radar than I do. It is as if they can literally feel a patient's inner pulse. Yet, other less effective doctors too often doubt the instincts of nurses, as well as of patients. Trying to convince a patient that everything is fine when he or she does not feel well is one of the worst things a doctor can do. It is an injustice, confusing and confounding the patient and leading to missed diagnoses.

When a patient suddenly becomes afraid that something is wrong and tells his doctor of his concern, a doctor should take this very seriously and assume that the problem is real. Fear is a primitive instinct emanating from the amygdala, an almond-shaped organ buried deep in the center of the brain. We inherit our fear instinct from our animal forebears, and when we respond appropriately, fear is part of our early warning system against danger.

Our inner pulse is informed by our deepest emotions, including fear. We can be alerted that something is wrong with our bodies, a powerful form of radar, long before a supposed expert tells us that we do or don't have a problem.

11

The Truth about Psychic Healing

If it's the Psychic Network, why do they need
a phone number?

—*Robin Williams*

Psychic healing has been practiced for centuries, and, when truly effective, it involves a contact with the inner pulse. It is wise to have an open mind with regard to the potential benefit of working with a gifted psychic. Some psychics are clearly quacks and charlatans, whereas others are true healers who have a window into the pulse. A true psychic may not only have the uncanny ability to predict when a person is becoming ill or is on the verge of death, but, when he is most effective, a psychic may exert direct influence to help keep a person alive.

In the mid twentieth century, Harry Edwards, a celebrated British healer (a printer by trade), worked by placing his hands on the

affected part of a patient's body. He started "healing" in his for-
ties, when several mediums informed him that he had the gift.
He reportedly cured a young girl with tuberculosis by simply putting his hands on the girl's head (he claimed that a sudden rush
of energy shot down his arms and into the patient).

Psychic healing was also carried on at a distance. Edgar
Cayce was born in Kentucky in 1877 and worked as a salesman
until age twenty-one, when he reportedly discovered that he was
able to cure his own laryngitis by willing his body to increase
blood flow to his voice box. Afterward, Cayce advertised his services, received names and addresses of new patients, put himself
into a trance, named the cross streets on his "mental" journey to
the patient's address, and was supposedly able to envision what
was wrong with the person by the time he "arrived."

Cayce believed that the cells of the body are individually conscious and communicate their condition to the larger spirit. This
notion is in keeping with my concept of the inner pulse. Cayce
gave close to ten thousand patient "readings" in his lifetime and
died in 1944 from exhaustion.

English psychic Matthew Manning claimed to be able to kill
cancer cells by touch and concentration and to improve many
medical conditions. This concentrated force, if it was real, apparently corrected a weakening in the inner pulse that would have
led to death. Doctors who observed the patients whom Manning
treated reported close to 100 percent improvement after the
treatment.

In parts of Asia and South America, psychic healers are often
accompanied by so-called psychic surgeons. Filipino psychic surgeon Alex Orbito has treated more than a million people, including actress Shirley MacLaine and Saudi royalty. Born in 1940, he
began healing at the age of fourteen, when he reportedly cured a
neighbor who was paralyzed. In 1999, Orbito built the Pyramid of

Asia Spiritual Healing Center in Cabanbanan, Manaoag, where he has been overwhelmed with eager customers.

Here in the United States in the 1990s, Anthony Fuina, a retired firefighter, claimed that he was miraculously cured by the touch of the famed healing priest Saint Padre Pio, thirty years after Padre Pio died. When Padre Pio reappeared, he supposedly put his hands on Fuina's belly and infused his supernatural power to strengthen and heal a failing inner pulse, thus curing Fuina's cancer. This story helped Padre Pio become Saint Padre Pio.

Here's how the story went: in 1997, Fuina, who was then sixty-two, was diagnosed with a bleeding precancerous tumor in his colon. Fuina said to me in an interview that his doctor (Dr. Ferrara) removed half of the tumor and planned to "go after the other half at another time."

"But then my wife received an *angel on the stoop*," he said. "My niece delivered it to my wife in a box as a belated birthday gift."

This was a sign that a personal miracle was about to happen, Fuina said, infusing power into his inner pulse.

Soon afterward, Fuina was driving and stopped for a bearded stranger. Fuina told me that the man was dressed in "clothes with squares in it, rough material, a white speckled baker's uniform." Fuina said that the stranger passed up a chance to get in two other vehicles that were waiting ahead of his car. "He waved to me and came right over to my car. He said, 'You have a medical problem.' He got in my car and prayed over me in tongues and laid his hands over me. I got goose bumps. He placed his hands right over the spot where my surgery was, at the bend of the colon, and there was heat in his hands."

The stranger then asked to be taken to the nearby Maria Regina church.

Later, when Dr. Ferrara operated on Fuina again to retrieve the other half of the tumor, he couldn't find it. "It was clean," Fuina said.

Three years later, in 2000, Fuina was diagnosed with cancer again—an incurable tumor of the esophagus. "It was in the wall of the esophagus," he said, "attached to the stomach, in the lymph nodes and had spread to the aorta." Fuina was operated on and received radiation and chemotherapy. "I received no burn marks from the radiation and lost no hair from the chemo."

His daughter handed him a small picture given to her at a prayer group where she was praying for her father. Fuina said that the photo, of Saint Padre Pio, looked exactly like the hitchhiker Fuina had picked up and who had laid a healing hand on his chest. Yet Padre Pio, who was known in his life for being in two places at once, had died in 1968, almost thirty years before the healing meeting with Fuina.

In August 2000, Fuina suddenly had no sign of cancer. "He had very advanced esophagus cancer," his radiation oncologist, Dr. Mitchell Karten of Nassau County Medical Center, told the *New York Daily News*. "His chances of being cured were very very remote."

As I observed the powers and the abilities of those outside traditional medicine, I learned that the inner pulse presents itself in different ways, depending on the context; that the inner pulse is a supreme force, as well as a path or a directive. It is the source of transcendence that can manifest itself as dying or as recovering health. It is a central power that a psychic healer can tap into.

Not all psychic masters who see inside us and claim to be able to influence what I call the inner pulse are authentic, but some are. I was learning to tell the difference. I want to tell you about one self-professed healer who truly puzzled me, and I wasn't able to tell whether he was real or fake, whether he was grandstanding or truly had his hand on the inner pulses of those he claimed to help.

When I was first contacted over the Internet by the self-proclaimed psychic Desmond Darrel in January 2009—after he'd heard me talking about health care on a popular overnight radio show—my first instinct was not to believe him. He seemed like a huckster who could hardly afford his storefront and was trying to drum up business through the Web.

Yet over time I began to reconsider. We had many e-mail exchanges that gradually impressed me. Although Desmond clearly didn't have any specific medical knowledge and barely understood how the organs of the body worked, he often had insights and foreknowledge that were hard to dismiss. As he zeroed in on my health and focused on keeping me and my wife well, I began to consider his comments relevant and look forward to his treatments through cyberspace.

What he referred to as "the energy" is comparable to what I call the inner pulse. He lived in Idaho, was seventy years old, and had worked as a psychic for thirty years, solving missing persons and murder cases, or so he said, claiming to "reunite the victim spirit with the family so it can move on and bring closure."

Desmond wrote to me that he had first noticed his ability by accident but had soon learned to control it. "What I do is first of all raise the energy levels in the body. Then I direct healing energy to the area that is most afflicted—lungs, heart, kidneys, pancreas, prostate, etc. I can measure the levels psychically. I can do this over the phone or the Internet."

Like many psychic healers, Desmond believed that his ability came from God, and that, empowered by God, one person's energy could affect the energies of the people around him or her. He said that in one case he found a draw of energy on a friend's wife and daughter and explained that, even if he raised their energy levels, he found that they would quickly drop again. Desmond did a psychic reading on all of the family's living relatives and found that the mother of the wife, who had emphysema and was dying, was acting as a draw and both her daughter and granddaughter were giving their energy to her without realizing it. Desmond said he started working on the woman and raised her energy levels so that her lungs improved from his measurement of 5 percent to 30 percent in two days. Once he did that, the drain was off the family and their energy levels stayed consistently high.

Desmond wrote that he was able to give energy to others without sacrificing his own. This is what he claimed made him an effective healer. In my terms, he was able to draw from his inner pulse without draining it. He supposedly gave strength to the inner pulses of those he healed.

Desmond said he helped out performing exorcisms at a church but that few knew of it.

He claimed to prefer to "fly below the radar." The town's sheriff's department had no record of Desmond working on missing persons or murder cases, as he'd claimed to do, but he had also said that these interventions were "two to four years after the fact" and did not involve the police directly.

Overall, I was not inclined to believe Desmond's wild claims that he could sense a person's "energy level" and that in general, death occurred below 20 percent, and healing occurred when he could bring a person above 70 percent. In fact, I was just about sure that Desmond was a phony until the day when he directed his e-mails toward my health, and then I became amazed at his perceptiveness, his seeming awareness of my inner pulse, and his apparent ability to strengthen it.

He sent me an e-mail one day indicating that he had done a reading on me from the picture on my Web site. My energy level was supposedly normal at 70 percent, but my lung readings were low at 10 percent, indicating that I might have a respiratory infection or asthma. Desmond was right about that; I was just recovering from a respiratory virus. He also reported my liver at 30 percent, which was below average and might be an indication that I took a medication that affected the liver. This was true, too, because I had been on Lipitor for several years.

"Your body gift is creative writing," Desmond wrote. "You folks live in a world all your own. The only way to make contact is for you to read it or for someone to write it to you. This can be a real problem in relationships. You have another gift, one of the seven gifts of the Holy Spirit. The gift of Faith. When people read your work it gives them faith. It looks like you have found your calling. I have only encountered about seven people in my life who have one of the Gifts of the Holy Spirit the way you do."

As I read Desmond's e-mail, I became suspicious again. Most of us want to feel that we have a special spiritual quality that Desmond was claiming I had. Was he trying to ingratiate himself to me so that I would believe he had special powers? It was certainly easy enough to conclude from my Web site list of publications that I communicated primarily by writing.

Two days later, Desmond wrote to me to say that my lungs had improved 30 percent, which had taken "some doing" on his part. He also took this opportunity to let me know that his readings could save patients and insurance companies on medical costs, and that he was available to speak at authors' groups or at readings I gave. This comment irritated me and again alerted me to the possibility that he was a scam artist.

He wrote to me again the following night. In addition to recommending goldenseal, echinacea, and "odorless garlic" for my cold, which he felt still hadn't resolved (he was right), he added that my kidneys were down to 30 percent, a sign of the cold itself or that my body was fighting back against it. I should drink more fluids, Desmond wrote—standard advice, although the notion of the kidneys being involved in fighting a respiratory virus was not something a traditional doctor ever believed.

I found this notion appealing, especially when I considered that the inner pulse did not obey specific organ boundaries but flowed equally through all of our organs.

If Desmond was a huckster, it was also seeming to me again that he had some real psychic abilities and a feel for the inner pulse. He was mercurial and flexible, didn't have set ideas, and was frequently prescient. This was appealing. It was as if he were paralleling the unpredictable waves of the inner pulse itself.

Early in the morning of January 29, 2009, Desmond wrote that my spirit had contacted him at 2:29 a.m. the night before. "All of a sudden I felt this movement of air right above my head— it was stronger than most contacts," he wrote. "I called your name in the form of communication I use. It responded. It did not tell me any secrets and I did not ask. I did a psychic reading on you to see if it was any different. The second was a reading on your wife. Her energy level was 40 percent—below normal. I will go to work on this."

Desmond was very concerned that my wife's kidney readings were only at 10 percent. He felt that the reading was most accurate because he was "working off a spirit that visited me in the night." He told me to look for puffiness in my wife's cheeks or lower back pain, where the kidneys are. Desmond wrote that he would be working day and night to bring my wife's energy levels up and help her kidneys.

Desmond's reading on my wife was uncanny, and I was immediately convinced that he had a feel for her inner pulse. For one thing, she had had a congenital kidney abnormality since birth, although her kidney function tests had always been normal, and for another, she had been feeling fatigued lately. Her face was often puffy from allergies. I found myself hoping that Desmond's healing energy would help her grow stronger, even if there wasn't a true health crisis in her life.

During the next few days, Desmond sent e-mails that he was working on my wife's energy levels and had them up to 80 percent and her kidney levels to 26 percent. If she didn't notice any appreciable difference in her energy levels, it was because our young child, Sam, continued to wake her up in the middle of the night.

On the other hand, as I began to exercise regularly, running on my treadmill and feeling stronger, Desmond noted that my heart energy was increasing. I developed a sore throat and treated myself with antibiotics, and Desmond reported that my kidney levels went up. Even if I didn't totally believe his assessments, his readings were becoming an unexpected supplement to my own sense of my inner pulse.

It is clear to me that psychic healers have a crucial role in reading the inner pulse. Many people have benefited from the insights and the interventions of true psychics.

Was Desmond for real? It was difficult to tell—but he did sometimes appear able to tap into the inner pulse.

PART THREE

The Pulse of Power

Your life is something opaque, not transparent, as long as you look at it in an ordinary human way. But if you hold it up against the light of God's goodness, it shines and turns transparent, radiant and bright. And then you ask yourself in amazement: Is this really my own life I see before me?

—*Albert Schweitzer*

12

The Strongest Inner Pulse

> No performer should attempt to bite off red-
> hot iron unless he has a good set of teeth.
> —*Harry Houdini*

The greatest performance artists and magicians appear able to bend and shape and focus their inner pulses to the point where they can accomplish feats that would seem to be supernatural or not humanly possible. Knowing your inner pulse and having a profound ability to control it may be the key to performances of extreme endurance and apparent magic.

Harry Houdini, widely recognized as the greatest magician and endurance artist of all time, was born Ehrich Weisz in Budapest, Hungary, in 1874, before emigrating to the United States two years later. He performed on a trapeze as early as age nine and began his career as a magician at New York's Coney Island amusement park at age seventeen, assuming the name Houdini in honor of his idol, the French magician Robert Houdin. Houdini soon became an expert at escaping from handcuffs and became famous in 1900 after handcuffing himself around a pillar at Scotland Yard and then breaking free. Among his most amazing stunts, Houdini escaped from the prison cell that held the assassin of President James Garfield; wriggled out of a strait-jacket while hanging upside down, and swam free of a crate that had been nailed shut and immersed underwater. As part of his regular act, Houdini would have himself placed in chains, completely submerged in a large container of water. While holding his breath, he could usually escape in only three minutes but would wait longer to create more suspense for the audience.

How was Houdini able to perform these feats? He trained relentlessly and pushed himself to his mental and physical limits. He practiced constantly, pushing his inner pulse until he had extended his ability to perform beyond what seemed humanly possible. He developed his capacity to hold his breath underwater by persistently testing himself in a very large bathtub he had installed in his house, seeing how far he could go before he drowned.

Houdini was anything but a psychic. He believed in God but strongly opposed the so-called spiritualists who claimed to be in contact with the dead and to be capable of performing feats of magic on that basis. Houdini's understanding of what I call the inner pulse was much more physical.

On the other hand, Houdini's friend Sir Arthur Conan Doyle, the creator of Sherlock Holmes, believed in spiritualism and was convinced that psychic powers enabled Houdini to perform his feats and escapes. Doyle was a proponent of what I might call the spiritual power of the inner pulse, although Houdini, his friend, vehemently disagreed.

David Blaine is an American magician and endurance artist who has deliberately fashioned himself in the style of the remark-able Harry Houdini. Blaine was born on April 4, 1973, half a century after the great man's death in 1926. Blaine seems to have developed the ability to focus his inner pulse as much as any man or woman alive. In my eyes, he is the new Houdini. Blaine emulates Houdini's continual pursuit of ever more difficult tasks and daring escapes.

Blaine performed magic tricks during his entire childhood. He taught himself to levitate and became famous at age twenty-four when ABC-TV produced a special called *David Blaine: Street Magic*. In 1999, he performed his first unprecedented feat, overcoming a fear that the great Houdini had always had—of being buried alive. Blaine buried himself underground for seven days at Trump Place in New York City without food or water, fueled only by his powerful inner pulse. The following year, Blaine froze himself in a six-ton block of ice in Times Square for sixty-one hours. This event was also featured in a live television special.

By the time I met David Blaine on a February afternoon in 2009 at his office/workout center in the Tribeca area of downtown Manhattan, he had accomplished many such seemingly impossible feats of endurance. At thirty-five, he was still in the prime of his career and was constantly reinventing himself in ways that would impress the great master Harry Houdini.

It was not surprising that I had to gain access to Blaine's office by solving a puzzle of turns and back-alley approaches. The neighborhood was a jumble of businesses and small residences, boutique shops mixed with lofts. I made my final right turn into an alley in between the buildings. Halfway down the alley, there was a small, unadorned, swinging iron gate, which was not locked.

Blaine spent his time training in a secluded office, one level down from the street. I arrived there for our meeting at 4 p.m. By the time I left two hours later, I was so entranced by the intensity of the interview that I found myself fumbling with the latch to let myself out.

His physical appearance was not imposing, although he was quite tall, well over six feet. I was able to tell him apart instantly from the other two magicians who worked with him by the intensity of his gaze. It was as if his eyes were direct beaming extensions of his inner pulse. I told him that I wanted to speak to him about how he was able to push himself into realities that defied science, guided by the force inside him.

He smiled, comfortable with the topic. We sat at a wooden dining table beneath an imposing picture of Houdini. David was spinning a bottle suspended by wires from the ceiling, with a playing card inside the bottle. He was trying to line up the card at a certain angle for the video camera that was filming him.

Afterward, he ate slices of skinless baked chicken and broccoli while we talked. He appeared deceptively simple. Rubbing his beard and staring straight ahead, he was defined by his intense concentration. I knew that at thirty-five, he would soon experience a fading of his ability to perform feats of pure physical prowess. As with Houdini, it was the physical, rather than the spiritual, aspects of what I call the inner pulse that interested Blaine the most. He compared the difficulty of his feats, saying that his forty-four-day hunger fast in 2003, when he lost 24.5 pounds, wasn't nearly as hard of a challenge as holding his breath on the *Oprah* show in 2008 for more than seventeen minutes underwater.

He was most proud of the letter he'd received from Dr. David Posner, a New York City pulmonologist who had examined Blaine beforehand and declared that he would never be able to hold his breath for a prolonged period, in part because of his small lungs. The letter was posted on Blaine's Web site. Posner wrote, "After giving it a great deal of thought, I have concluded that I don't think we can make David Blaine look like he's not breathing under water for 20 minutes. Since expired air only contains a few percentage points of carbon dioxide, one cannot help but need to move at least 5 liters of air per minute in and out of the lung, and this is having a person hypoventilate. . . . By the way, he doesn't have very big lungs, with his TLC (total lung capacity) being only 80% of predicted. . . . People can't fly, and they can't breathe under water. . . . So far, it appears that Mr. Blaine's illusions have all pushed the limits of normal human endurance. None of them have rewritten physiology."

When I spoke to Blaine in his office/training suite, it was clear that he agreed with Posner in one respect: his breath-holding episode was by far his greatest challenge and the only challenge that completely rewrote expectations about physiology. For this reason, it was also far more interesting to him (and to me) than anything he had ever done, before or since. There was never an issue of making him "look like he's not breathing," the way Posner nastily insinuated. For Blaine, his performance was never about appearance or simulation; it was real. His goal was to push past the realm of what was perceived to be humanly possible.

I believe Blaine may have as much command of his inner pulse as anyone alive. Before appearing on *Oprah* in April 2008, Blaine shattered the world record of holding his breath underwater (which had previously been 16 minutes, 32 seconds). "I held my breath for twenty minutes," he said. Yet Blaine felt that the appearance on *Oprah* was more difficult. "I was nervous. I had trouble keeping my heart rate down."

Blaine's heart rate, which rose to more than 40 beats per minute on the *Oprah* show and included irregularities and frequent extra beats, caused his body to burn more fuel and require more oxygen than even his prior 20-minute episode. The fact that he held his breath for 17 minutes, 4 and 4/10ths seconds, in a water tank on *Oprah* was simply unbelievable and one of the most incredible feats of defying physiological limits ever accomplished.

"It was unnecessary for me to train all of the time in preparation," Blaine said. "The key was to role model others who had accomplished similar things. I spoke with the record holders, who had held their breath for sixteen minutes. They gave me techniques. But no one was more of a role model for me than the great Houdini."

Blaine ate carefully while we spoke, chewing every morsel of food several times before he swallowed. He said that while he was in training, he was "treating my body as a machine," guided by the "wholesome, energy-driving, fat-burning energy" advice provided by a nutrition program designed for professional cyclists. He rarely went out and didn't socialize. He lived a simple, directed life.

"Food is my medicine," Blaine said. "I look for nutritional impact, the exact nutrition I need to do the job."

In each part of his preparation, Blaine willed himself to go beyond his stated goals, relying on his ultra-powerful inner pulse as he directed and conditioned his body.

"I've been training my whole life," he said. "Working on willpower."

Blaine had trained for the breath-holding event by swimming, running, jumping rope, and practicing holding his breath for at least two hours each day, much as Houdini had. "One key is being around people with the same thoughts as you every day, people who believe you can do it. I set a simple goal for myself that I can understand and surround myself with those who support my goal."

The inner pulse thrives in an environment of positive thought and emotion. As Blaine strove to surpass the other breath-holding champions, he gently discounted what Dr. Posner had warned about. Blaine said he realized that rigid doctors might not know someone's limits, and that they would always hedge on the side of what they knew to be safe.

"Someday we will have the technology to predict this. A doctor will be able to hook a person up to a computer and tell him what he can do. It will free doctors up to think more. In the meantime, a doctor has to be cautious, to play it safe. I understand that."

I didn't think medical instruments would ever be able to successfully measure the inner pulse, but I did believe that the technology of the future might be better at sensing it.

No doctor today would predict that a person could hold his or her breath for twenty minutes, Blaine said. "One day they will be able to. Doctors told me that if I held my breath for twenty minutes, my brain will lose oxygen and I will die. With computer advances, a doctor will have more information to guide whether it's okay or safe for a particular person."

While Blaine was training for his breath-holding ordeals, he drank no alcohol. He worked on expanding and focusing the force within him and didn't allow it to be weakened by negative distractions. As he readied himself for *Oprah*, he held his breath for fifteen minutes and had a vascular surgeon check him out—the doctor was amazed at the fact that Blaine could still think clearly at the conclusion of the episode.

Blaine trained for *Oprah* for four months, following two years of longer-term practice. "I was willing to die for my goal," he said nonchalantly.

Yet when he finally got there and was down in the tank underwater, as he approached seventeen minutes, his heart rate got away from him. It sped up, and he had an irregular rhythm; he could feel sudden death coming on him. He could feel his body ending, reaching its physical end, and he pushed it; he could feel the inner pulse stretched to its natural limit.

"Because I was prepared, nothing was going to stop me. My heartbeat was irregular, I knew I could stop it. I was going into cardiac arrest, I stopped it. You feel your body. How close to the edge you are."

For Blaine, this was his most spectacular feat ever. He didn't consider his hunger fast for forty-four days in London in 2003 to be in the same category. He considered the fast a great experience of the spirit, a "heightened sense of awareness through deprivation." Blaine acknowledged the spiritual side of the pulse more than Houdini did, but like Houdini, Blaine's most impressive work involved the sheer power of channeling his great abilities to overcome physical impossibilities.

David Blaine sees his life through the prism of someone who knows his own body, repeatedly challenging the limits of his own inner pulse. "It's a matter of personal hunger," he said. "The body gets your signals. Houdini was the hungriest. He laid the groundwork."

Blaine said that Houdini's great mastery was a combination of talent, willpower, and knowledge. Blaine acknowledged that he was patterning himself after the supreme escape artist. "I try to work hard," he said, "to resist the offers of the world. If the challenges are great, then the results are not tricks. It is a desire that comes from within."

Why was he able to accomplish these nature-defying feats of endurance and seeming magic when others were not? I asked.

Blaine answered humbly. "All people are really capable of the same things," he said.

I told him I didn't agree. A consummate mind-body champion such as Blaine or Houdini was one of a kind. No one else came close.

Blaine smiled; his eyes glittered with the confidence of his accomplishments. He deeply understood that he'd been born with an unprecedented ability to focus his inner pulse, the way a magnifying glass can focus sunlight and make fire from it.

Believing in God made him humble and grateful for his gift. He had unique and prodigious skills, but he told me he knew that they emanated from a far greater source.

Although very few of us indeed can channel our inner pulses to the same, almost miraculous extent as Blaine, all of us can learn from his example, and we can all extend our capabilities.

13

Who Dies? Who Lives?

> There was now a partial glow upon the fore-
> head and upon the cheek and throat. A per-
> ceptible warmth pervaded the whole frame;
> there was even a slight pulsation at the heart.
> The lady *lived*.
>
> —*Edgar Allan Poe*

Just when I think I can sometimes predict a disease's deadly
outcome by recognizing a patient's inner pulse, someone comes
along to remind me how much I still don't know—how much we
all still don't know.

Todd Barnes was a poet, a playwright, and a lyricist. He
worked in relative obscurity for most of his life, despite the
fact that he collaborated with famous artists. Todd wrote librettos for operas and converted short stories into plays. His own
poetry remained largely unknown but stayed in print with a small
California press. His greatest play, a romantic tragedy, is still
being performed on college campuses.

I first met Todd in the winter of 1993 at the Century Club in
Manhattan, having been invited to a concert. I was introduced to

Todd at the bar. When he heard I was a physician, his tone turned serious, like that of someone who had rehearsed his responses to doctors. He told me that he no longer drank alcohol but missed the bar scene, so he stayed near the bar at parties.

Todd said he was looking for a new doctor and asked me for my business card.

The writer Kurt Vonnegut walked past, smoking a cigarette, and overheard us. "Oh, doctors," Vonnegut said, waving his arms. "Keep them away from me." Vonnegut died of lung cancer a few years later.

The following spring, Todd came to see me in my office. He slouched when he walked. He wore loose-fitting clothes and talked in easy slang.

In the examination room, he mocked his short, backless cloth gown, flashing a toothy grin that seemed out of place with the medical circumstances. Yet the instant he turned to discussing his health, he became serious.

"I think I have a serious problem that other doctors have missed," he said, worried. "I hope you are thorough."

I was becoming used to patients feeling changes in their inner pulses before the doctors who treated them were aware of anything amiss. Sure enough, I discovered that Todd's liver tests were slightly elevated, and I tested him for hepatitis. It was right about this time that the first blood assay for hepatitis C had become available, and Todd's test came back positive. This was the first diagnosis of hepatitis C that I had made. His ultrasound showed that his liver already had the beginnings of cirrhosis, permanent liver damage. I sent him to a liver specialist, who suggested the antiviral treatment alpha interferon, which was the only drug in use for hepatitis at that time. The treatment made Todd feel very fatigued and flu-ish, and he quickly stopped it.

Todd continued to come to me as a patient, and our friendship began to flourish outside the office. We sometimes met for dinner at at an old Mexican restaurant downstairs from the hotel where he lived. The fish stew was rich and salty, like Todd's personality.

At the height of our friendship, we sat around the hotel smoking cigars dipped in brandy, and Todd handed me a folder full of his poems and plays. I was particularly interested in his dramatic rendering of one of Chekhov's stories, *Ward Six,* in which Dr. Ragin, a physician, becomes so disillusioned with society that his only remaining friend is a paranoid schizophrenic who is interned in an insane asylum. Dr. Ragin gradually loses everything and is committed as a patient in the same hospital, whereupon his only remaining friend turns against him.

In 1996, as Todd began to succumb to liver failure, his bloodstream filled with toxins that affected his brain, a condition known as hepatic encephalopathy, and he required larger and larger doses of a synthetic sugar, lactulose, which draws the liver toxin ammonia from the blood. There were times when he was completely awake and alert, but at other times he was confused, despite the medicine. Whenever I spoke with him on the phone and he sounded groggy, I urged him, "Have a swig of your magic elixir."

At the same time that Todd's mental and physical faculties were deteriorating, I entered a stage in my life comparable to Chekhov's Dr. Ragin. As I mentioned, I became anxious, in part as a result of the stress of a new marriage; my first novel, *Bellevue,* which was about to be published; and my first son, Joshua, who was soon to be born. Even after his birth, I often woke up in the middle of the night, worried that my new son might stop breathing at any time.

Todd knew I was suffering. I didn't share the details of my metaphysical confusion and pain with him—I tried to focus on his disintegrating liver and how to compensate for it with diuretics, in addition to the lactulose. I kept working and I managed to keep making unexpected diagnoses, and in one of my best moments, I instinctively sent Todd for an ultrasound of his abdomen, although he was feeling well at the time. The ultrasound showed a mass in the liver.

Looking back, I realize that I had been directed by a sudden intuition that something was wrong with Todd's inner pulse.

I feared that I was too late. Masses are large punctuation points in medicine. They automatically instigate a complicated work-up and often result in a disastrous diagnosis. Todd's was such a case—his liver biopsy revealed hepatocellular carcinoma or hepatoma, primary cancer of the liver. Although there was no evidence that this nasty cancer had yet spread, the five-year survival rate for this type of cancer with conventional chemotherapy was only 4 percent.

I immediately suggested a liver transplant, but, after first considering it, Todd refused. "I know I won't survive it," he said.

He also claimed that Medicare would never approve the operation because of his hepatitis C, a destructive virus that could recur after the transplant. Todd's new oncologist, Dr. Jean Francois, agreed that Todd should have the transplant. Dr. Francois also believed that Medicare would not pay for it. Todd's wealthier friends began to raise money for the operation, but before they reached the needed $100,000, Todd told them to stop. He had decided against the operation, no matter what.

I couldn't get him to change his mind, and the more I pushed him, the more I feared I would lose him as a friend. I was just beginning to learn to defer to a patient's strongest intuitions and feeling for his own proper path.

Todd chose a liver specialist at Mt. Sinai, a direct competitor of my hospital, claiming that our top expert had mistreated his friend, a famous painter, by accepting a priceless painting in return for a few five-minute visits. The painter ultimately died of the same cancer that had long gone undetected.

Yet Todd was grateful for my quick diagnosis, and in addition to his new liver specialist, he continued to see both me and Francois.

In the summer of 1997, we admitted Todd to my hospital's co-op care section, a 1970s hotel-like facility that was becoming obsolete in the 1990s amid shrinking reimbursement rates. Todd had decided to try a new kind of treatment known as chemo-embolization. Pioneered by Dr. Judah Folkman, this technique involves administering chemotherapy through the artery that feeds the tumor, then destroying the artery. This treatment was revolutionary in the 1990s; it is now used for more than one million patients in thirty-plus countries, although it does not generally cure liver cancer. Back in 1997, no one knew how effective it would be.

When Todd nervously entered the co-op care unit, the last thing he was expecting at 11 p.m. the night after his first treatment was a frantic call from his doctor, waking him from sleep.

"I think my wife is going to leave me," I said.

"I think your wife is a wonderful woman. Do you also wake her up in the middle of the night?"

I paused, suddenly embarrassed that I had called Todd so impulsively. Why had I done so? I was supposed to be the one taking care of him, and he had just received an experimental chemotherapy treatment. I had considered the proximity of his bed across the street a comfort. He was close by, a familiar voice in the middle of my sleepless night, and he was often awake late at night and had sometimes even called me after 1 a.m. Yet, of course, he was a sick patient. I had no such excuse.

Afterward, I felt awful. Todd kept me as a physician, although he never stopped reminding me of the inappropriateness of that call. He began to see me as more selfish and less reliable.

Miraculously, Todd and I began to heal simultaneously, as if our inner pulses were both benefiting from the contact. His tumor shrank in response to the treatment, and although I kept waiting for the mother tumor to regrow and shoot its metastatic tentacles around the body, his follow-up CT scans and MRIs continued to be negative.

Unfortunately, the hepatitis C virus continued to eat away at his liver, and he stubbornly refused further traditional antiviral treatments.

"Enough of poisons," Todd said. Instead, he turned to a maverick physician, Emanuel Revici, who was one hundred years old and still practicing alternative medicine. Years later, Todd would credit the Revici purges and enemas and mystery combo chemicals for prolonging his life, rather than the single chemo treatment he had undergone, which had likely produced benefits for only four or five months. He would receive only one further chemo-embolization years later, whereas the Revici treatments remained a steady part of his routine for years.

Born in Romania in 1896, Revici began on the traditional side of medicine, receiving his medical degree from the University of Bucharest in 1920. He practiced internal medicine, while researching lipids and cellular metabolism. He wore thick, dark glasses, which, together with his conservative suits, gave him the look of a serious scientist. He moved to Paris in 1935, then to Mexico City in 1941, where he began to experiment with drugs to treat cancer.

Professional cancer societies began to consider him anything but a scientist. Revici came to New York in 1947 and started

the Institute of Applied Biology, where he continued to conduct experimental cancer research. A study published in the
Journal of the American Medical Association in 1965 revealed that
of thirty-three patients who were referred to Revici after they
failed conventional treatment, twenty-two died, eight showed
no improvement, and the remaining three showed progression of
their disease. Yet Revici continued to expand his treatments. In
the 1980s, he received more than seventeen patents for chemical
formulations to use on cancer patients.

He remained extremely controversial. According to an article
in *Cancer Journal for Clinicians* in 1989, New York State challenged and restricted his medical license, finding him guilty of
professional misconduct in 1988. Investigative reports have stated
that his license to practice medicine in the state of New York was
revoked in 1993.

Todd met Revici in 1997, when he was one hundred years old
but still advising his treatment group. Todd was very impressed
with Revici's philosophy of healing and his convictions that cancer was due to an imbalance of fat in the body, which he supposedly determined by analyzing a patient's urine. Todd was also
drawn to the fact that Revici's treatments involved mixing a soup
of disparate ingredients, similar to the way Todd approached
writing. Revici's "guided chemotherapy" often included a secret
formula made of alcohols, caffeine, zinc, lithium, iron, selenium,
magnesium, sulfur, and/or fatty acids.

According to Todd, Revici also looked deeply into Todd's eyes
to study his tormented soul and figure out a personal concoction to
heal it.

"You have to meet him. Then you'll take him seriously," Todd
said. He arranged a dinner for us to exchange ideas, which I readily agreed to, but the medical heretic, who was spry and vital until
his last days, died of a sudden heart attack a few days before the

meeting was to take place. After his death, Todd and many others continued to receive treatment at his center.

Meanwhile, I was regaining my equilibrium, step by painful step. As I wrote in chapter 1, I was able to cure my anxiety by holding on to my small family, to my one-year-old son. I slowly began to feel more anchored. I began to monitor my emotional reactions to people and spent more time with people whom I felt good with and less time with those who made me feel bad.

What Todd and I had in common, in terms of our healing, was that both of us held fast to our deepest intuition and belief in ourselves.

Todd survived against all odds. He continued to come uptown to see me at monthly intervals. Looking at his bloated belly on the examining table, feeling his swollen ankles, and smelling the ammonia-laced breath that stemmed from his liver failure, I sometimes found it difficult to believe that he really was in remission, and yet, as the years went by, he remained cancer-free. He continued to credit the Revici purges and enemas and mystery combo chemicals for prolonging his life. He altered his diet dramatically, forgoing heavy, salty Mexican meals in favor of salads, fruits, and pasta.

Was it possible that the effect of a single chemo-embolization treatment had lasted so long? Responses were unpredictable, and genetic factors were crucial in this response. Tumors might look the same from the outside, but they could arise from variations in many different genes, making them more or less responsive to drug A, drug B, or drug C. A study from the Broad Institute of MIT and Harvard, published in 2008 in the *New England Journal of Medicine*, reported a genetic pattern in liver tissue that correlated with survival and lack of recurrence of liver tumors. Some patients were very sensitive to certain treatments, based on their genetic makeup. Not all practitioners who explored the effects of genetic variance on treatments used accepted principles of science. Dr. Stanislaw Burzynski, a pioneer to some and a heretic and a quack to many others, was a believer in combination gene-targeted therapies, focusing on the "genetic signature" that was unique to each cancer patient. He was the discoverer of antineoplastons, treatments with a genetic basis that targeted cancer but hadn't really been proven to work.

Between 1998 and 2005, Todd worked on several librettos, refusing to think of himself as a sick person with spreading tumor cells. "The force is with me," he often joked. He believed that as long as he kept working, he would stay alive, as if he could influence his inner pulse to keep him safe. Perhaps he did. I also saw writing as Todd's therapy and was convinced that the passion for his work that kept burning in his mind helped keep him alive.

Did Todd have a genetic predisposition toward remission? In all studies of cancer, there are some patients who simply survive no matter how grim the prognosis. Unfortunately, patients such as Todd fuel the myths of the heretical healers of the world such as Revici without providing any real evidence to support their fringe treatments. I would never actually recommend the Revici treatments to anyone, although Todd thought that I would.

Even as he remained alive, after 2002, Todd grew more and more bitter and began to withdraw. The cancer was gone, but the hepatitis C virus was still active, damaging his liver and poisoning his body. Toward the end, in 2005, as he dipped deeper and deeper into a virus-induced encephalopathy that fogged his brain, he began to lose track of our friendship and to see me only as the troubled doctor who had called him once in the middle of the night back in 1997.

This distancing from his doctor and friend had waxed and waned, just as his reaction to his failing liver had waxed and waned. I blame myself for blurring the distinctions between physician and friend that allowed Todd to alternatively embrace me and reject me.

In late 2005, when Todd was finally admitted to the local VA hospital for a serious infection and out-of-control diabetes, he didn't want to see me or most of his other close friends and doctors. He was transferred to a hospice, where he soon died.

Obscured in the unpleasantness of his dying was the miracle of his cancer remission. Ten years after he was diagnosed with cirrhosis and eight years after developing terminal liver cancer, it was not Todd's liver that finally killed him.

There is little scientific evidence that a patient who conceives of himself as healthy can more easily remain so, that a patient refusing to succumb to his illness has his mind working for him rather than against him. Science notwithstanding, however, my experience as a physician has taught me that it is sometimes true. Would science ever catch up to this possibility? In Anne Harrington's *The Cure Within* she tracks the holistic health community's seizing on cancer as being "a wake-up call from the body that makes clear just how steep is the price for all these too common failures of personality and courage."

Of course, acknowledging that stress and worry can contribute to cancer is not the same as proving that personality or courage can cure it. Susan Sontag famously protested against this type of thinking in her 1978 book, *Illness as Metaphor*.

Dr. Bernie Siegel disagreed. In 1986, he wrote in his book *Love, Medicine, and Miracles* that cancer was a challenge to people that he could help them face. Unfortunately, a follow-up study of Siegel's patients published in the *Journal of Clinical Oncology* in 1993 found that women with breast cancer who went through his mind-body program died at the same rate as those with breast cancer who hadn't. Evidently, simply thinking positively didn't grant automatic access to a healing inner pulse.

Todd Barnes was a study group of one—his cure was not scientific proof that positive thinking helps keep you alive longer. It may have contributed in Todd's case and in mine, but in the end we both owed our comebacks directly to something more essential, something we all have deep within us that we can learn to rely on.

14

Considering the Alternative

The voyage of discovery lies not in finding new landscapes but in having new eyes.

—Marcel Proust

Susan O'Hara, a sixty-four-year-old woman, had been diagnosed with breast cancer in 2000. She was treated by the alternative healer Dr. Ben Miller, who had a strong belief that Susan could avoid a recurrence of her tumor after a lumpectomy by changing her lifestyle, taking up relaxation techniques, and undergoing herbal and hormonal treatments. In Susan's case, at least, he turned out to be right. She told me later that she had a powerful sense of her inner pulse being strong and healthy—she never thought that the early cancer would recur or become life-threatening—which is why she had sought out Miller rather than sticking with a surgeon or a more traditional oncologist.

"Her back was against the wall," Miller told me dramatically. "At first, I didn't think she'd make it."

Miller was a tall, thin doctor in his mid-forties. He was known for his flashy brand of charisma. He had perfect teeth, and he liked to chew gum. He had trained in traditional medicine (psychiatry) but had forsaken it for a more holistic approach.

He believed in preventive medicine and herbal treatments, and although I was very concerned about his eagerness to dispense active chemicals and hormones, including testosterone and estrogen, I also felt that his ideas about rejuvenation and antiaging made some sense. Miller and I were friends, and he sent patients to me for more traditional treatments.

After treating Susan for her breast cancer, Miller referred her to see me. I would be her regular internist. Susan was very thin, weighing 113 pounds at 5 feet 3 inches tall, although she said that she'd maintained the same weight for years. She had a strong family history of breast cancer: both her sister and her mother had also developed breast cancer in their sixties. Susan had undergone a lumpectomy but resisted further treatment. She told me that she was worried about recurrences but was against the idea of "poisoning" her body with chemotherapy or radiation. She had seen Miller because he offered her another way.

She was very happy with the results and was a big advocate of his brand of medicine. He had treated Susan with a combination of glucosamine, calcium, vitamin C, zinc, branched-chain amino acids, carnitine, melatonin, a secret protein formula called "brain mood," B-complex vitamins, niacin, co-enzyme Q10, omega-3 fatty acids, flaxseed oil, fish oil, alpha lipoic acid, pregnenolone, aspirin, urocitrate, vitamins A and E and C, NA cysteine, tryptophan, and 5 mg of testosterone. Susan had apparently responded.

"Testosterone and progesterone were once used to treat breast cancer before they had these new chemotherapies," Miller said.

He claimed that her cancer had recurred before his treatments.

When I reviewed Susan's records, I wasn't as sure that the hormones were the cause of her cure, and I could find no evidence whatsoever that her cancer had recurred. Her breast biopsy from 2000 did not show extensive disease but rather a very small—some would say—precancerous lesion known as ductal carcinoma in situ. She had had it removed surgically, and although the tiny tumor was high grade, poorly differentiated, and extending almost to the surgical margins (signs of aggressiveness), many of these tiny tumors did not return.

The tests he'd ordered—ultrasounds, mammograms, and MRIs of the breast—continued to show that Susan's breasts were clear of disease. Did Miller's treatments play a role in Susan's happy outcome, or was the relationship between treatment and cure serendipitous? It was difficult to tell.

It was certainly clear to me that Miller felt he had helped cure Susan, and it was also true that he was more mindful of what I call the inner pulse than many traditional doctors would have been.

Miller had a kind of magnetism that drew patients to him. Some patients were so committed to Miller's charm and array of treatments that they repeatedly returned to him. He had a deep empathy. Even if I objected to many of his treatments and felt that he often went too far, I also believed that many traditional doctors did, too.

Alternative treatments are very popular, although it is difficult to prove how effective they are. The National Center of Complementary and Alternative Medicine of the NIH reported in 2005 that $19 billion was spent on alternative treatments in the United States, two-thirds of it paid for in cash, and that 62 percent of Americans were using some form of complementary and alternative medicine (CAM). Were these treatments effective? Did they alter spiritual and physical wellness by affecting the inner pulse? The answer is that some did and others didn't. Some of these healers were pretenders, while others had great insights and treatments. It was often difficult to tell the difference.

In 2007, biostatistician R. Barker Bausell, the former director of research at a center for complementary medicine at the University of Maryland, authored *Snake Oil Science: The Truth about Complementary and Alternative Medicine*, in which he maintained that therapies as different from one another as acupuncture, chiropractic treatment, herbal medicine, hypnosis, and energy healing all have one thing in common: they make people feel better by virtue of the placebo effect. The treatments may work, but they do so at least partly by the power of the mind influencing the inner pulse. To be sure, herbal treatments have proven medicinal value, but *belief* in a treatment adds to this value.

In *Snake Oil Science*, Bausell proposed that by appearing to be caring, alternative providers often convince patients that questionable treatments really work. These so-called healers get false credit for the natural waxing and waning of an illness, determined by the inner pulse. Patients tend to remember their initial symptoms as being worse than they really were, which makes CAM seem even more effective. This is not to say that there is no place for alternative approaches or that they don't reach or influence the inner pulse. In fact, the alternative methods that are most effective and true have an impact on the pulse. Whereas the concept of the inner pulse is overlooked by a narrow, rigid, traditional approach and is not part of the medical school curriculum, the concept of something akin to the pulse is central to spiritual healing, even if the healer doesn't use the term per se.

The Cleveland Clinic recently completed a complementary and alternative therapy pilot program for patients undergoing heart surgery, where half of the patients opted for art, music, or touch therapy; guided imagery; or spiritual guidance. Almost 100 percent found the services helpful.

In addition, herbs, when used properly, can have great medicinal value and can stimulate the inner pulse. The legitimate study of the properties of herbs traces back to ancient times. Just to name a few, according to Chris Kilham, the famous Medicine Hunter: Cat's claw, the root bark from an Amazon vine, works well as an anti-inflammatory and an anti-allergy treatment. Rhodiola rosea, a plant that grows in cold regions of the world, including northern China, boosts energy and mental acuity. The goji berry is good for vision and overall health, and the maca root, which comes from the Peruvian highlands, is well-known as an energizer and a libido stimulator. A healer may consider these herbs fuel for the pulse.

Some alternative healers can effectively combine serious science with spiritual healing. Dr. Shem Altman is one such serious scientist. He is a clinical, anatomical, and chemical pathologist by training. He has successfully converted his background as the former medical and laboratory director for SmithKline Beecham labs into a career as a medical investigator and an alternative healer. He is an expert in dealing with complex cases that defy traditional attempts at diagnosis.

In the 1990s, Dr. Altman worked in emergency rooms in Georgia and urgent care centers in Florida, honing his skills at clinical problem solving. He began to work with toxins and cellular injury and the immune impairment that results from chemicals in the environment, as well as from radiation, inflammation, and the effect of viruses. He examined what happens when the natural DNA-driven repair mechanisms no longer work, and the resulting immune dysfunction leaves the body vulnerable to disease.

In his detoxifying treatments, Altman attempts to "reduce the cellular injury that caused the problem in the first place." Altman routinely treats patients with damaged livers and cancer due to hepatitis. "It is a race against the clock," he said to me, "between reducing tumor burden and restoring healthy physiology."

Although Altman began to work with detoxification in New York, he found that he was limited by New York State law, which restricted his laboratory testing. He moved to Scottsdale, Arizona, in 2007 and began to offer a comprehensive analysis of elements found in the body, such as toxic metals and nutritional minerals in the hair, the blood, the urine, and the feces, as well as other organic toxins that have a more chronic and insidious effect. The inner pulse is negatively affected by these toxins, and a patient's health is jeopardized. Altman agrees with my concept of the inner pulse as the body's spiritual and physical fulcrum and says he believes that when he is successful at detoxifying the body, he affects the inner pulse in a very positive manner.

Altman is committed to his patients and keeps in close touch with them. "I detoxify people and help them restore their physiology," he said.

Altman has made many important discoveries, including the fact that heavy metals such as rubidium can cause anxiety, emotional instability, insomnia, fatigue, and increased pain. He has also found that increasing zinc in the diet can help people overcome the effects of mercury toxicity. Altman thinks that the food we eat often lacks the trace elements we need. Even more problematic, according to Altman, our vegetables and fruits "pick up whatever elements are in the soil where [they] is grown."

Altman is a physical chemist for the immune system. His goal is to repair the damage that toxins do to the body and indirectly to the mind. His work has a very strong and positive impact on the inner pulse. He is not as self-promoting or as grandiose as Miller is, but his results are more verifiable and often more dramatic. The two doctors share a recognition of the importance of the inner pulse, although their methods for stimulating it are very different.

With the inner pulse, there are many roads to healing.

15

Miracles and the
Inner Pulse

> Demons do not exist any more than gods do,
> being only the products of the psychic activ-
> ity of man.
>
> —*Sigmund Freud*

From the moment Father Matthew Pell first came to see me in 1999, he was anxious about his health.

Pell often didn't feel well and was frequently frustrated by medical science's inability to help him. He was always concerned that he might be dying, but he really wasn't dying. Even though he was a man of God and quite effective spiritually with members of his parish, he seemed incapable of knowing his own inner pulse—which resonated with life and sometimes with illness, but not with impending death.

In 2005, Pell was admitted to the hospital where I work with mysterious abdominal pains that led to an extensive negative work-up. I can still picture him standing in the middle of his room, pointing to his stomach and gesticulating wildly with his arms. "I'm not well," he said. "There's something terribly wrong with me."

Two days later, he grudgingly went home, complaining bitterly at the inadequate nursing care and the fact that no definitive result had been found. Pell was deceptively soft-spoken and reassuringly polite, but he was also relentless in his complaining.

There were actually several reasons for him to feel ill, even if he lacked the life-threatening diagnosis that he so anticipated. He had emphysema from smoking, congestive heart failure, and hepatitis C.

For his hepatitis he saw another doctor, with a name similar to mine, who practiced gastroenterology at a hospital downtown. This doctor had a very different approach to Pell's hepatitis than I did. He wasn't aggressive, didn't order liver biopsies, and didn't offer treatment.

"What are we going to do if we find cirrhosis?" the doctor asked when I called him.

"Treat him with antivirals," I replied.

"He won't tolerate it," he insisted. We were getting nowhere. Pell liked both of his doctors, while I disliked the gastroenterologist who resembled me in name only. Over the years, Pell went to see the other doctor less and less often, not because he was taking my side of the dispute, but in an effort to consolidate his care under one roof.

One day in November 2008, he sat before me, appearing anxious. "I know something's wrong," he said. "Something awful."

I looked at him closely. Was his inner radar alerting him, or was he just nervous? I had learned that even patients who were prone to false alarms might still achieve moments of clarity and insight when, all at once, they sensed their inner pulses. It was always foolish and bad doctoring for me to be dismissive of a patient's complaint. "What is it?"

The troubled priest rose slowly from my blue couch. What was he about to do?

"Sit down, sit down," I said anxiously.

"Are you ready to listen to me?" he asked.

"Always."

He then told how he had been losing weight for the last few weeks, that his hips and knees were killing him, that his orthopedist was trying a new kind of pain injection that wasn't really working, and that he slept very little because of the pain. "What should I do?" he asked.

I suggested a new sleeping pill or anti-anxiety medication, but Pell waved his arms at me and barked, "That's all you do is throw pills at me."

"If you aren't feeling well, I will find out why," I vowed.

"It's too late for that," he said. He stood, wobbling unsteadily at the door to my office, his shakiness due to a combination of pain in his joints, Parkinsonian balance problems, and early dementia. Seeing him in so much physical difficulty, yet at the same time trying to dismiss me without provocation, I felt frozen and ineffective.

I followed him to the elevator and stridently tried to talk him into coming back, but he wouldn't reconsider and fled down in the elevator.

After he left, I sat at my office desk and tried to compose myself. I cared about Pell, despite his cantankerousness. His chest X-ray was hanging on the X-ray view box. I stared at it uncomprehendingly until I gradually realized that it wasn't normal. Each X-ray has a characteristic array of pulmonary vessels, lung, and sometimes scar tissue that identifies its owner. Pell's X-ray had always been dark from emphysema and trapped air (air is black on an X-ray), but today there was something new, a round shape with a jagged edge located in the middle of the right lung.

Coupled with Pell's recent weight loss and fatigue, I suddenly became worried that he might have cancer. Maybe he was another Kahn, in touch with the radar of his inner pulse. All of his complaining was a smokescreen for this sudden alert. He knew it, but I had missed it. I felt terrible. How was I going to communicate my concern to him now that he had left my office? He needed a CT scan of the lungs as soon as possible to help determine what the lung mass was.

I left him a message on his answering machine at the church, saying that I needed to speak with him as soon as possible. Cancer was like a personal terrorist, and the thought of it pushed people into a deep cycle of worry. Pell was bound to be frantic.

I called the general number at the church where Pell was the pastor and spoke to his assistant, who was also a patient of mine. He said he would tell Pell to call me immediately.

Finally, I called Pell's psychiatrist, Dr. Blatt, and told her what had happened. Blatt assured me that she would reach Pell and make sure he had the CT scan and would try to convince him to return to me.

I remained distressed. A patient with a possible cancer, an inner pulse that was alarming him—this was the worst time for there to be a rift in a doctor-patient relationship. Yet right now, there was nothing else I could do about it.

Have you ever noticed that after you handle a situation poorly, something else immediately goes wrong to pay you back? I tend to believe that we live in a spiritual world of karma, connected through everyone's inner pulse. For physicians who deal with intense life-and-death matters on a daily basis, payback often seems to occur right away.

The same night that Pell stalked out of my office, seven hundred miles away in Michigan, in what felt like punishment for my lack of sufficient sensitivity with Pell, my father-in-law, Alex, with his eyesight failing from many years of poorly controlled diabetes, took the wrong dose of insulin. He was soon lying on the floor of his bathroom, unable to move. My mother-in-law, Tamara, fully paralyzed except for one tremulous arm from two decades of multiple sclerosis, couldn't reach the med alert button that my wife had had installed over their bed.

Tamara spent the next hour trying to reach for the phone, which was on the blanket just beyond her grip. Lying inert, she finally managed to move the blanket just enough to get the phone to roll toward her (it could just as easily have rolled away). She telephoned her son, thirty-eight-year-old Moshe, a soft-spoken six-foot, six-inch man who wore the top hat and the *peyis* of the *frum*, or Orthodox Jew.

Moshe, a computer engineer who was impoverished by the basic needs of his nine children, drove the short mile between his small ranch house and his parents' apartment. Reaching the fourth floor, he lumbered to their apartment, and, finding the door still locked, he broke the door open with a single push of his shoulder. His parents had a health aide throughout the day, but the aide had left ten minutes before Alex's mistaken injection. Seeing his father lying on the floor, Moshe lifted him up onto his shoulder, then called 911. The ambulance arrived ten minutes later. By this time, Moshe had called us in New York, and my wife, a neurologist, had come to the conclusion that her father had suffered a stroke.

Luckily, EMS protocol proved otherwise. Responding by rote, they injected Alex (or Papa Sasha, as we called him) with a concentrated sugar solution, and he instantly responded, becoming more alert and slowing regaining sensation and movement in his legs. It seemed clear to the attendants that he had a low sugar level from an overdose of insulin.

It was 1 a.m. The EMS techs placed an intravenous line in my father-in-law's arm and carried him out of the apartment on a stretcher, with Moshe following. Tamara was left alone with the phone now in her hand, waiting for her aide to arrive in a few minutes to spend the rest of the night.

The events that followed seemed anything but random, which is often the case when only the inner pulse is left between life and certain death. One minute Sasha seemed about to die, the next minute it looked like his life wasn't at risk at all. He was brought to Beaumont Hospital in the suburbs north of Detroit. I had never heard of Beaumont. In the past, Sasha had always been taken to city hospitals, where his foot infections had been slow to heal and his shortness of breath too often ignored. At Beaumont, however, the ER doctor quickly determined that my father-in-law had sustained some heart damage—his cardiac enzymes (troponin) were slightly elevated. He also had an irregular heart rhythm (atrial fibrillation), although, luckily, he was now no longer weak on one side.

I decided to fly to Michigan. I would do my best to reverse any bad karma and to help Papa Sasha.

I arrived later that morning. Sasha was admitted under the care of Dr. Steve Ipsen, whom he had seen once a year earlier. Ipsen, a cardiologist who specialized in invasive procedures, was urging a cardiac catheterization (in which a catheter is fed up to the heart through the groin, and blocked coronaries are ballooned open and kept open with stents).

I called Ipsen from my rental car. He told me he would perform the procedure the following morning. Yet I still had to convince Moshe, who would then convince his father that the catheterization was necessary. I explained that the small heart attack meant that there was a partial blockage, and stents might help keep a more serious heart attack from occurring.

Moshe, however, looked for direction from the writings of the Rambam, Moses Maimonides, the sage physician and prophet from the thirteenth century whom I've discussed earlier in this book. Maimonides had proposed that there were times when intervention or healing was indicated, whereas at other times the body was simply declaring itself with symptoms. Healing would often occur without a procedure.

Sasha wasn't religious like his son, but, like his son, he was trained as an engineer and understood immediately as I explained how stents worked. Father and son agreed to the procedure for different reasons, and it was scheduled for the following day.

In the morning my wife, Luda, called me frantically while I was still at my hotel. Ipsen had flown out of the country to Germany for a conference without notifying us, and Moshe had just learned that Ipsen had asked his junior associate to do the procedure.

"Let me see what I can find out," I said to my wife.

I called Dr. Fred Feit in New York, the director of our own cardiac catheterization laboratory at the time and a prominent pioneer in the world of coronary angioplasty. Fred had been my friend for many years. He was a very thin, jocular man approaching sixty who still appeared athletic. He ate sparsely, mostly potatoes; was on good terms with the people who hadn't pissed him off; and often acted far more humbly than his credentials warranted.

"Fred, I'm here in Detroit, and my father-in-law has had a small heart attack. The guy who was supposed to do the catheterization just left for Germany. I am uneasy about letting his young associate do it."

Fred was the first to agree that medicine—especially, this procedure—was a fine art, depending entirely on the skill of the artist.

"Where are you? What hospital?"

"A place in the middle of nowhere called Beaumont. Has a lot of nurses. But how good can it be?" I said.

"Beaumont?" Fred chuckled. "Middle of nowhere, you say? You happened to land at one of the top two or three heart hospitals in the country. That is the place to be. Cindy Grines has been the head of the lab there for several years. She is one of the best in the world. She has conducted many of the major studies. She's at least as good as I am. Tell her I told you to call. I will also call her myself."

Fred knew his own worth. For him to say that another interventional cardiologist was as good as he was—this was significant.

At the mention of Fred's name, Cindy Grines rearranged her busy schedule to take the case. A few hours later, sitting with Moshe at my father in-law's bedside while he said one prayer after another, I reconsidered a notion that Richard Sloan put forth in chapter 9 of this book—that prayer, per se, doesn't influence medical outcome.

Ipsen's unexpected last-minute trip to Europe had resulted in my phone call to Fred, which had led to the discovery that we had a better choice available for a doctor. It all seemed like a tiny miracle, rather than just a coincidence.

When Dr. Grines approached us with a serious, yet breezy manner right after the procedure, I was sure that Moshe's prayers had been answered. Grines looked to be in her early fifties, her thin athletic face showing a few wrinkles. "Two tight lesions in the left anterior descending artery," she said. "The rest is mild disease. We opened the arteries and gave him two Cypher (drug-coated) stents to keep them open. He'll do fine."

Moshe and I were quite relieved. We had never gotten along well in the past, but we were now becoming friends. We viewed the spiritual and scientific intersection that had saved his papa the same way. The science had saved him; the coincidences had optimized his chances.

Back in my office in New York on Friday morning, Jasmine told me that Father Pell had gone for the CT scans I'd ordered. It was irrational, especially given the horrible-looking lesion on his X-ray, but I now had the strong feeling that the scan would turn out all right. Pell's inner pulse had alerted him to a problem, but now the spiritual winds were at our backs, and our collective karma had improved. I called the radiologist—the pipe-smoking Alec Megibow—to see whether Pell's CT scan report was back yet, and he told me that he would have the results in an hour. While I waited, I reviewed all of Pell's X-rays from the previous five years with my office mate, the pulmonologist Dr. Adams. Looking at each one closely, he was able to determine that the mass had been there before, although it seemed to have grown. Cancer seemed less and less likely.

The day had the texture of coincidence to it. Diagnoses were coming in clusters: two patients in a row had draining pustules on their buttocks that needed to be lanced, followed by two with pneumonia in the same part of the lung. David Hume, the naturalist philosopher, would likely have said that I was so focused on these coincidental clusters when they happened that I tended to miss the unremarkable background of unconnected diagnoses that made up the bulk of my daily practice. Hume would have denied a supernatural event and called it a perceptual problem on my part.

Yet I was pretty sure Hume would be wrong, especially when two novelists in a row (both patients) came in with eyelid infections and I referred them to the same eyelid specialist, Dr. Palu, whom I hadn't had occasion to call for several years.

This particular Friday seemed to be a page torn out of the supernatural world. The patient clusters and their positive outcomes seemed like spiritual weathervanes pointing toward the direction of the future health outcomes of Pell and my father-in-law.

There were other coincidences that day, almost as if I'd entered a rift in time and space. I accidentally left my laptop—containing most of the chapters of this book—on a desk in the busy lobby of Bellevue Hospital. Hours later, it was still there, despite thousands of poverty-stricken patients passing by in the meantime. On returning to my office, I accidentally placed a folder for this book marked "Active File" in a pile of patient charts. Luckily, my office manager Jasmine had a hunch to show it to me just before filing it with the patient charts under the letter A.

"Did you misplace this?" she asked, not sure what it was. It included the notes for this chapter. It was a sign that my fortune had changed. Just as the sky was darkening with the oncoming Sabbath, I received the two phone calls I was hoping for. My father-in-law, Sasha, was now home in his own bed. And Dr. Megibow called to say that Pell's CT scan was negative. I immediately called the church. The assistant said he would give Pell the good news, and he said he was sure the priest would return to see me again.

For me, the shifting medical winds were no coincidence and were tied to the mitzvahs that I and others had done. They represented the connection that the inner pulse had with the greater spiritual world and showed how the direction of a health outcome could be changed by the right intervention—just as the great rabbi Maimonides had once written.

Do miracles take place in contrast to natural law, or are they ultimate manifestations of nature and an extension of the inner pulse we all have?

St. Augustine maintained that a miracle is not contrary to nature but only to our knowledge of it, that miracles are hidden potentialities in nature that are placed there by God. St. Thomas Aquinas said that a miracle must go beyond the order that is usually observed in nature, although at the same time a miracle is not really contrary to nature because it is ultimately a manifestation—like all things—of God's will.

In more contemporary times, R. F. Holland argued that a miracle is always consistent with natural law, emphasizing that a religiously significant coincidence may qualify as miraculous, even when we fully understand the causes that bring it about. Holland's views were very much in keeping with the principles of this book. Scientific understanding never compromises the power of the inner pulse and its many manifestations, and vice versa. David Hume, however, was dubious of many supposed miracles and did not believe that real miracles flowed from nature but only from God. He wrote that "no testimony is sufficient to establish a miracle, unless the testimony be of such a kind, that its falsehood would be more miraculous."

In the early twentieth century, Ludwig Wittgenstein saw miracles as simple signs that are in keeping with nature. Wittgenstein wrote, "A miracle is, as it were, a gesture that God makes. As a man sits quietly and then makes an impressive gesture, God lets the world run on smoothly and then accompanies the words of a saint by a symbolic occurrence, a gesture of nature."

Like Wittgenstein, I was starting to see miracles as simple extensions of God and of nature. I was aware of this in the events I'd experienced with my father-in-law, as well as with the priest. I think the Rambam (Maimonides) might have put it this way— the decision to proceed with Sasha's heart catheterization and to bring in the best possible practitioner available to save him had been a mitzvah, an action taken to restore his health, and had led to a sign that it was the right decision as Ipsen flew away in the middle of the night and Dr. Grines, a more qualified expert by far, was suddenly there to take over. This action, together with prayer, had come in the aftermath of my insensitive behavior with priest Pell. Yet in helping my father-in-law, I'd acted with a renewed spirit of healing that had then extended back toward Pell.

I felt God's presence as I learned my lesson through the evolution of several small personal miracles. Rabbi and prophet Lubavitcher Rebbe Menachem Schneerson had commented on the biological evolution of miracles when discussing the Torah section known as "Korach." In this section, the high priest Aaron, Moses' brother, has a staff that produces fruit and ripe almonds.

According to Rebbe Schneerson, God didn't simply make almonds appear; he stimulated the process of the emerging and ripening of the fruit. In this way Aaron's staff appeared to be defying natural laws, while at the same time conforming to them. The almonds' appearance transcended nature, but they grew and developed like real almonds.

Schneerson contrasted this kind of miracle with a "confrontational miracle," where the reality is completely contrary to nature's laws. Schneerson believed that a miracle that is integrated with nature is even more elevating than a miracle that supersedes nature. It is this kind of miracle that resonates most with the uncanny workings of the inner pulse. Brian Solomon's rising out of his wheelchair was a miracle, but it was a miracle in keeping with the natural medical world. The same was true for the great feats of David Blaine or the miraculous cures I've written about in this book.

Rabbi Schneerson was an inspirational teacher and healer. According to the mystical text *Tanya*, the use of religious words mediated by the great Rebbe sometimes led to bodily healing. *To Know and to Care* is a book of Chassidic stories about Schneerson and how people came to him for blessings, which ended in miracles. In one such story, painter and Russian rabbi

Chanoch Hendel Lieberman went to Schneerson feeling hope-
less about his stomach cancer, which several doctors had said
was terminal. Yet Schneerson advised him that if he found a doctor who was willing to operate on his stomach, he would survive.
Lieberman then managed to find such a surgeon and ended up
living for another eighteen years. Here was another miracle that
complemented rather than contradicted science.

Schneerson saw these miracles as God's response to acts of
kindness, when people who went beyond their innate self preoccupations were rewarded. They could also be seen as miracles manifested in the inner pulse, with Schneerson exhibiting great vision
in seeing the spiritual message inscribed inside a person's flesh.

Schneerson died in 1994 of a stroke. My wife, Luda, was a
beginning neurology resident at the time, and she took care of
him in the hospital during his last few months. People were visiting him from all over the world, talking constantly about his great
powers. They were sending notes and calling him by the hundreds, many begging him for one last miraculous blessing.

Yet the rebbe whom Luda saw was sick, paralyzed on one
side, too weak to leave his bed, not speaking, and despite all of
his great works and deeds, despite all of the blessings he'd given
and the medical miracles he'd witnessed, like all humans, he was
unable to commandeer one last miracle for himself.

Strengthening his failing inner pulse was beyond even the
great rabbi's ability.

Afterword

All in Good Time

The inner pulse is elusive. It lurks below the surface in all of us and has a direct link to our souls. The inner pulse cannot be measured, but we can learn to recognize it. In this book, I have tried to provide insights into how and when the inner pulse appears.

You can learn to interpret your inner pulse. You can receive direction from it: the inner pulse is your connection to the larger spiritual world. The inner pulse can teach you how to move toward better health, and, as it finally ebbs, it can also show you how to die.

Some of my patients are more in touch with their inner pulse than others are. I have learned to listen and to listen carefully.

You can choose healers by how attuned they are to your inner pulse. Some doctors can recognize the characteristic patter of the pulse; others can't. Learning how to sense the inner pulse is not a skill that can be strictly taught, but it can be acquired by a physician during many years of careful listening and observation.

To a biologist or a medical practitioner, death and dying do not always appear to be either moral or dictated on the basis of reward or punishment. I believe that God is present in the tiniest bacteria, as well as in the white blood cells fighting them. At the same time, twenty years of practicing medicine have repeatedly shown me that pneumonia and influenza kill old folks whether they are nice or nasty. Some of my patients have died right in the middle of their most profound observations. Many deaths occur at the end of a relentless march of an organism or a cancer that just can't be stopped, that can't be treated, willed, or prayed away.

There are times, though, when scientific explanations fall short of the actual situation at hand, when the only explanation lies with the spiritual and physical fulcrum that I call the inner pulse. The process of following the mysterious path of the inner pulse has led me into arenas as different from one another as mysticism and determinism are.

What is most striking about these cases is the way they are fueled by deep intuition that runs contrary to science and probability. In each case, someone—either the patient, a family member, or the doctor—has an unshakable belief that emanates from the inner pulse, tied to an uncanny, unexpected medical outcome.

Almost everyone, no matter how scientific his or her background, asks the same question—Why me?—when faced with a life-threatening illness. Even if we are completely rational all of our lives, illness automatically leads us to broaden our search. Few are stoic enough or linear enough in their thinking to accept biology as the total answer. "Why me?" opens the door to inquiries into philosophy, religion, and mind-over-matter medicine. "Why me?" is an opportunity to explore ancient mysteries, as well as the limitations of technology. Dr. Michael Gruber, a brain cancer expert at NYU, is one physician who believes that converting

"Why me?" into a more positive attitude is at least one potential factor in overcoming deadly cancer.

Attempts to defy the odds not only help patients face devastating diagnoses, they also help doctors attempt ambitious or even dangerous cures. Gruber's decision to give immunological vaccines and the solid-tumor chemotherapy drug Avastin to patients with terminal glioblastomas had been spawned by his courage to fight in the face of overwhelming odds.

Ambitious treatments that defy probability are not limited to cancer alone. Dr. Leon Pachter, the chief of surgery at my hospital, recently removed a gall bladder laparoscopically from an eighty-year-old patient of mine who was so frail and compromised by his heart failure and lung disease that an open surgical procedure would likely have taken his life. Sticking the laparoscope in through his navel and removing the gall bladder via this tiny incision was much less of a direct threat to his feeble medical condition, but because of the scars inside his belly from a previous operation, few besides our chief would have attempted to pass the scope.

Dr. Pachter, a deeply religious man, kept the negative odds in the background, while in the foreground he considered his patient's keen intelligence and his will to live. He performed a successful operation on a patient who had a very strong inner pulse. Afterward, the patient rapidly recovered.

Encountering Pachter at ten o'clock one night in the garage beneath the apartment building where we both lived, I asked him why he had attempted the risky operation. He had the reputation of being a very conservative surgeon. Had he sensed the man's indomitable spirit?

He shrugged. "I had a feeling that he was stronger than he looked. He's a tough old guy," he said.

"Did you know he was going to make it?" I asked him.

The chief was a man of few words. "I had a strong feeling," he said. Pachter had guts, and he relied on his instincts, essential qualities of a great surgeon. He had chosen to operate based on his intuition and faith that he could succeed—a decision made from the realm of the inner pulse, beyond the world of surgical science.

As I mentioned in the preface, my Polish Jewish great-grand-parents were killed by Cossacks in a pogrom. I always imagined that the frequent bouts of depression that my grandfather Alex suffered—he sat in a dark living room behind closed drapes for months after losing his job as a tool-and-die maker—were the direct result of his losing these precious parents at the age of thir-teen. The facts of our family's history afterward were well known to me—Alex's older brother, Abram, was already in the United States, so Alex, as the oldest son still in Europe, was left in charge of his sisters Paulie, Fanny, and Lena at the time of his parents' death. Lena was only nine months old and had barely survived a brutal clubbing from one of the Cossack murderers. The family came across to America by ship, and Alex went to work, starting several businesses before teaching himself the trade of tool-and-die making, while learning to speak and write in six languages.

My grandfather Alex was an atheist, and I suspect that the experience of the pogrom was the reason. It was always difficult for him to find a silver lining to things. In 1981, Alex was ninety-one, blind, and living in a nursing home when he developed a pre-leukemic condition. He was brought to the hospital for treat-ment, and while he was there, he contracted colitis (inflamma-tion of the bowel). My father, Bernie, authorized a colonoscopy, and the gastroenterologist punctured my grandfather's colon in the process.

He never really recovered after that and suffered through recurrent bouts of pneumonia. My father came to visit him in the hospital almost every night. One night, my father noticed that his father was looking better, acting more alert, and breathing a bit more easily. My dad felt guilty that the tests he'd sanctioned had led directly to Alex's downhill course, and he was glad to think that Alex was experiencing a reprieve. After half an hour of sitting with him, my father got ready to leave.

"Stay for a while," my grandfather said.

"I have to get home to my family," my father replied.

"You are a big disappointment to me," my grandfather said.

Bernie thought that his father was referring to his consent to all of the procedures on his father's behalf. Or perhaps it was a more pervasive dissatisfaction. Alex was never one to pull punches, and as he had gotten weaker and sicker, all of his son's decisions had seemed wrong. This negative cascade of events is familiar to any physician who treats extremely ill patients. It feels like an undertow dragging you and your patient down—it is difficult to reverse, guided by a negative force that is not completely explainable by science.

This undertow was the inner pulse weakening and fading. My grandfather knew it. He could feel his life force ebbing, even if there was no way to measure it. He had a premonition that night that he was going to die, and he wanted my father to stay with him. He told the nurse to tell Bernie, but the nurse had forgotten, and my father had returned home. Later that night, my grandfather developed a mucus plug in his lung, started coughing and gasping for air, and died a horrible death by asphyxiation. Afterward, my father said he would never forgive himself for not staying with his father.

I was in my first year of medical school at the time, and the story had a big impact on me. The inner pulse weakening was manifested in a patient's ability to know when he was dying even when science didn't predict it. I was alerted to this phenomenon at an early point in my training, and I began to study it. This was not about a son failing to say good-bye. It was about a father—Alex, who knew death intimately—knowing when his time had come.

In contrast to Alex's, Bernie's life has not been marked by tragedies. It is as if the family karma has changed. I've always felt that my mother was to thank for this. She is a cheery person who appears to have been rewarded for her generous nature by having her husband, my gruff father, accompany her to a healthy old age.

Watching my parents grow old has helped me learn to look to the inner pulse for the greater truth.

In August 1997, my father was seventy-three. Having recently witnessed the birth of his first grandchild, Joshua, my father awoke from sleep with chest pressure that wouldn't go away. He had already survived two previous balloon angioplasties of his coronary arteries (these angioplasties were performed in the era before Dr. Fred Feit and other interventionalists had tiny cylindrical stents to keep the arteries open). My father spent the night in the bathroom putting one nitroglycerin under his tongue after another, until, in the early morning, the pain finally subsided. Never wanting to bother anyone about his health, my father tried to go back to bed.

At 8 a.m., the pain returned, and he called me. When I heard what was happening, I told him to take another nitro, which took away the pain. I jumped in my car and drove out to Long Island at 90 m.p.h. The trip took half an hour, and I knew I was taking a chance. I should have called 911, but I also knew that if I did, he would be taken to the nearest hospital, where he had previously waited for hours in the ER for a prostate infection. I had a strong instinct—almost a premonition—against having my father go to the local hospital. Looking back now, I am sure that what drove me was a deep connection to my father's inner pulse. I didn't sense any weakening in his life force, and I was following my deepest intuition emanating from that force.

When I arrived at my father's house in East Meadow, Long Island, at 8:30, he was feeling better. The pain had returned briefly, he had popped another nitro, and the pain had gone away again (nitroglycerin dilates the coronary arteries that supply the heart, giving it needed oxygen). Now that I could grab his hand and stare at him sternly, I was able to convince him that he was at great risk. At the same time, I was even more confident in my intuition that he would ultimately be fine. I was ready to drive him to one of the better Long Island hospitals, which was only twenty minutes away and had a renowned heart program. Yet he refused to go there as well, recalling the time he had gone with severe back pain and had waited hours to be seen.

"They ignored me," my father said. "Everyone sits there waiting. Hangnails along with heart attacks." My mother quickly packed an overnight bag, and my father joined me in the car and insisted that we speed back to New York City. I tried again to convince him to go to a hospital on Long Island, but he refused.

As I was driving, I called my old friend Justin, a cardiologist on the faculty of three top Long Island hospitals. Justin said that he was in New Jersey and estimated that he could make it back to the hospital in a little more than an hour. My father liked Justin and trusted him but still preferred to take the risk of going to New York, especially since Justin wasn't close by. Justin would be phone-ready in case there was a problem. I also had a vague premonition that even though Justin was a well-trained, experienced cardiologist and a close friend, if I turned my father over to Justin's care, something bad could happen.

During the harrowing drive into the city, my father remained symptom-free. I knew that he could have a deadly heart arrhythmia, an irregular rhythm, from angina at any time. I was relying on my intuition and the fact that the abysmal family bad luck had changed since the day of Grandpa Alex's death. Driving my father into my hospital was the kind of jump into the unknown that more cautious doctors rarely make. Yet as I've discussed throughout this book, too many doctors lack a feeling for the inner pulse and the emotional momentum that results from it. At the conclusion of our successful trip, I felt as if I'd driven fast along a slick wet road without incident.

Dr. Feit and his team were there to receive us with skilled hands, just as Fred would be available to guide me exactly ten years later with my father-in-law. In 1997, it was found that my father's main artery (left anterior descending) on the front side of the heart had once again clogged with cholesterol-laden plaque. This time when it was reopened, a tiny metal stent was placed into the artery to keep it that way.

Bernie has been healthy ever since. Many times, I've revisited my decision to take the drive, instead of simply calling 911. It is unquestionable that the statistical risk of taking him into the city was greater than whatever the risks were of receiving treatment on Long Island. I was driven by intuition this time, rather than by science, and I believed the likelihood of a positive outcome depended on Bernie's strong inner pulse. It pushed him past the dangerous moments to a cure, and he has remained in good health ever since, even as many of his friends have died of cancer and heart disease.

The series of events that appears to have liberated the Siegels from our family legacy in Poland brings to mind Carl Jung's famous concept of synchronicity, which suggests a link between the mind and the world that resonates with a transcendental truth. Jung believed in "meaningful coincidences," when there is a connection between events that have a coincidence in time.

Justin's being out of town and my father's delay in telling me both improbably contributed to a successful outcome. Jung believed that the unconscious mind manifests in the world of perception: "the premise of probability simultaneously postulates the existence of the improbable."

My own struggles with anxiety were budding and peaking at the same time that my father became ill. Somehow I managed to control my worries just long enough to care for him. Afterward, I dissembled, even as he was healing and regaining his strength. My inner pulse was weakening, even as his was strengthening, as if the spiritual energy that was necessary to heal him had come from me.

More than a year later, when I regained my own bearings, the realization that my cure was within helped me immeasurably. I had the strong positive instincts I needed to help myself against the odds as my father had done.

I believe my resilient inner pulse comes primarily from my mother, and the more I follow it, the more it leads me away from being ill and back in the direction of being well.

During the course of my life and my medical career, I have learned to feel my way along, bypassing illness and returning to good health. In this book, I have tried to describe the insights I learned along the way so that you can apply them to your life, to your distinctive inner pulse, and to the healers you choose to help you find your way. There is no medical textbook to explain the inner pulse, and there will never be one, but I often feel that I helped keep my dear father alive because I learned to follow in good time the spiritual path to good health.

I wish you good health as well.

Bibliography

Preface and Introduction

Bowman, Deborah, and Daniel Sokol. "Secrets and Lies." Student *BMJ* 9, no. 2 (2009): 50–51.

Brann, Eva. *Feeling Our Feelings: What Philosophers Think and People Know.* Philadelphia, PA: Paul Dry Books, 2008.

Chopra, Deepak. *The Book of Secrets: Unlocking the Hidden Dimensions of Your Life.* New York: Three Rivers Press, 2005.

———. *Reinventing the Body, Resurrecting the Soul: How to Create a New You.* New York: Crown Archetype, 2009.

———. *The Seven Spiritual Laws of Success: A Practical Guide to the Fulfillment of Your Dreams.* San Rafael, CA: New World Library/Amber-Allen Publishing, 1994.

Dispenza, Joe. *Evolve Your Brain: The Science of Changing Your Mind.* Deerfield Beach, FL: HCI Books, 2008.

Duffin, Jacalyn. *Medical Miracles: Doctors, Saints, and Healing in the Modern World.* Oxford, UK: Oxford University Press, 2008, 5, 7, 17, 31, 35, 37, 40, 71, 74, 99, 111, 113, 115, 122, 123, 128, 129, 142, 144, 154, 171, 179.184, 189, 190.

Freud, David, and Linda Freud. *The Healing Gift: Exploring the Remarkable World of a Medical Intuitive*, 1st ed. Laguna Beach, CA: Basic Health Publications, 2010.

Freud, Sigmund. *The Uncanny.* New York: Penguin Classics, 2003.

"From Kishineff to Bialystok: A Table of Pogroms from 1903 to 1906." Museum of Family History, www.museumoffamilyhistory.com/ajc-yb-v08-pogroms.htm.

Fulford, Robert, DO. *Dr. Fulford's Touch of Life: The Healing Power of the Natural Life Force.* New York: Pocket, 1997.

Hammond, Kenneth R. *Human Judgment and Social Policy.* Oxford, UK: Oxford University Press, 1996.

Hawking, Stephen, and Leonard Mlodinow. *The Grand Design.* New York: Bantam Dell, 2010.

Hogarth, Robin M. *Educating Intuition.* Chicago, IL: University of Chicago Press, 2001.

Kleinman, Arthur, MD, MA, Leon Eisenberg, MD, and Byron Good. "Culture, Illness, and Care: Clinical Lessons from Anthropologic and Cross-Cultural Research." *Annals of Internal Medicine* 88, no. 2 (February 1, 1978): 251–258.

Louise, Rita. *The Power Within.* Seattle, WA: BookSurge Publishing, Amazon.com, 2002.

Meier, Diane E., MD, Anthony L. Back, MD, and R. Sean Morrison, MD. "The Inner Life of Physicians and Care of the Seriously Ill." *JAMA* 286 (December 19, 2001): 3007–3014.

Melchizedek, Drunvalo. *Living in the Heart: How to Enter into the Sacred Space within the Heart.* Flagstaff, AZ: Light Technology Publishing, 2003.

Oates, Wayne E. "The Inner World of the Patient." *Pastoral Psychology* 8, no. 3 (1957): 16–18.

Pintoi, Angelo J., and Howard J. Zeitz. "Concept Mapping: A Strategy for Promoting Meaningful Learning in Medical Education." *Informa Healthcare* 19, no. 2 (1997): 114–121.

Regan-Smith, M. G., S. S. Obenshain, C. Woodward, B. Richards, H. J. Zeitz, and P. A. Small Jr. "Rote Learning in Medical School." *JAMA* 272, no. 17 (November 1994): 1380–1381.

Royle, Nicholas. *The Uncanny.* Manchester, UK: Manchester University Press, 2002.

Schulz, Mona Lisa, MD, PhD. *Awakening Intuition: Using Your Mind-Body Network for Insight and Healing.* New York: Three Rivers Press, 1999.

————. *The Intuitive Advisor: A Psychic Doctor Teaches You How to Solve Your Most Pressing Health Problems*. Carlsbad, CA: Hay House, 2010.

Siegel, Marc. "Putting Extra Care into Health Care." *Washington Post*, May 1, 2007.

Warner, Marina. *Phantasmagoria: Spirit Visions, Metaphors, and Media into the Twenty-First Century*. New York: Oxford University Press, 2006.

Weil, Andrew, MD. *Spontaneous Healing: How to Discover and Embrace Your Body's Natural Ability to Maintain and Heal Itself*. New York: Ballantine Books, 2000.

1. Surgeons of the Mind

Conway, Jim. *Men in Midlife Crisis*. Colorado Springs, CO: David C. Cook, 1997.

Diamond, Stephen. "Normalcy, Neurosis and Psychosis: What Is a Mental Disorder?" www.psychologytoday.com/blog/evil-deeds/201003/normalcy-neurosis-and-psychosis-what-is-mental-disorder, March 11, 2010.

Frankl, Viktor E. *Man's Search for Meaning*, Cutchogue, NY: Buccaneer Books, 1993.

Gaudette, Pat. *How to Survive Your Husband's Midlife Crisis: Strategies and Stories from the Midlife Wives Club*. New York: Perigree Trade, 2003.

Hart, Archibald D. *The Anxiety Cure*. Nashville, TN: Thomas Nelson, 1999.

"Humor Therapy." American Cancer Society, www.cancer.org/Treatment/TreatmentsandSideEffects/ComplementaryandAlternativeMedicine/MindBodyandSpirit/humor-therapy, accessed June 11, 2010.

Jacques, Elliot. "Death and the Midlife Crisis." *International Journal of Psychoanalysis* 46 (1965): 502–514.

Kruger, A. "The Mid-Life Transition: Crisis or Chimera?" *Psychological Reports* 75 (1994): 1299–1305.

Lachman, Margie. "Development in Midlife." *Annual Review of Psychology* 55 (2004): 305–331.

Lachman, Margie, ed. *Handbook of Midlife Development*. Hoboken, NJ: John Wiley & Sons, 2001.

Lad, Vasant. *Ayurveda: A Practical Guide: The Science of Self Healing*. Twin Lakes, WI: Lotus Press, 1993.

Myers, David G. "Adulthood's Ages and Stages." *Psychology* 5 (1998): 196–197.

Sheehy, Gail. *Passages: Predictable Crises of Adult Life*. New York: Dutton, 1976.

Siegel, Marc. *Bellevue, a Novel*. New York: Simon & Schuster, 1998.

———. *False Alarm: The Truth about the Epidemic of Fear*. Hoboken, NJ: John Wiley & Sons, 2005.

Whitbourne, Susan Krauss. *The Search for Fulfillment: Revolutionary New Research Reveals the Secret to Long-Term Happiness*. New York: Ballantine Books, 2010.

2. The Pulse of Recovery

Bassetti, C., F. Bomio, J. Mathis, and C. W. Hess. "Early Prognosis in Coma after Cardiac Arrest: A Prospective Clinical, Electrophysiological, and Biochemical Study of 60 Patients." *Journal of Neurology, Neurosurgery, & Psychiatry* 61, no. 6 (December 1996): 610–615.

Blackmore, S. J. "Near-Death Experiences: In or Out of the Body?" *Skeptical Inquirer* 16 (1991): 34–45.

———. "A Psychological Theory of the OBE." *Journal of Parapsychology* 48 (1984b): 201–218.

Blackmore, Susan. "Out-of-the-Body, Explained Away, but It Was So Real . . . *The Archive of Scientists' Transcendent Experiences, TASTE*, www.issc-taste .org/arc/dbo.cgi?set=expom&id=00075&ss=1.

Blakeslee, Sandra. "Studies Report Inducing Out-of-Body Experience." *New York Times*, August 24, 2007.

Blanke, O., S. Ortigue, T. Landis, and M. Seeck. "Stimulating Own-Body Perceptions. *Nature* 419 (2002): 269–270.

Booth, C. M., R. H., G. Tomlinson, and A. S. Detsky. "Is This Patient Dead, Vegetative, or Severely Neurologically Impaired? Assessing Outcome for Comatose Survivors of Cardiac Arrest." *Journal of the American Medical Association* 291, no. 7 (February 18, 2004): 870–879.

Chen, R., C. F. Bolton. *Young BCrit Care Med*. "Prediction of Outcome in Patients with Anoxic Coma: A Clinical and Electrophysiologic Study." *Critical Care Medicine* (April 1996): 672–678.

Chow, E., T. Harth, G. Hruby, J. Finkelstein, J. Wu, and C. Danjoux. "How Accurate Are Physicians' Clinical Predictions of Survival and the Available

Prognostic Tools in Estimating Survival Times in Terminally Ill Cancer Patients? A Systematic Review." *Clinical Oncology (Royal College of Radiologists)* 13, no. 3 (2001): 209–218.

Christakis, Nicholas A. *Death Foretold: Prophecy and Prognosis in Medical Care*. Chicago, IL: University of Chicago Press, 2001.

Christakis, Nicholas A. and Elizabeth B. Lamont. "Extent and Determinants of Error in Doctors' Prognoses in Terminally Ill Patients: Prospective Cohort Study." *BMJ* 320, no. 469 (February 19, 2000).

Coma Information Page. National Institute of Neurological Diseases and Stroke, www.ninds.nih.gov/disorders/coma/coma.htm, accessed June 12, 2007.

D'Souza, Dinesh. *Life after Death: The Evidence*. Washington, D.C.: Regnery Press, 2009.

Ehrsson, H. Henrik. "The Experimental Induction of Out-of-Body Experiences." *Science* 317, no. 5841 (August 24, 2007): 1048.

Glare, P., K. Virik, M. Jones, M. Hudson, S. Eychmuller, J. Simes, and N. Christakis. "A Systematic Review of Physicians' Survival Predictions in Terminally Ill Cancer Patients." *BMJ* 26, 327(7408) (July 2003):195–198.

Jauhar, Sandeep. "The Instincts to Trust Are Usually the Patient's." *New York Times*, January 5, 2009.

Jung, Carl. "1944: Sick Bed Visions." In *Memories, Dreams, and Reflections*. New York: Pantheon, 1963.

Kaplan, P. W. "Electrophysiological Prognostication and Brain Injury from Cardiac Arrest." *Seminars in Neurology* 26, no. 4 (September 2006): 403–412.

Lenggenhager, Bigna, Tej Tadi Thomas Metzinger, and Olaf Blanke. "Video Ergo Sum: Manipulating Bodily Self-Consciousness." *Science* 317, no. 5841 (August 24, 2007): 1096–1099.

Levy, D. E., D. Bates, J. J. Caronna, et al. "Prognosis in Nontraumatic Coma." *Annals of Internal Medicine* 94 (1981): 293–301.

Long, Jeffrey, and Perry, Paul. *Evidence of the Afterlife: The Science of Near-Death Experiences*, 1st ed. New York: HarperOne, 2010.

Meili, Trisha. *I Am the Central Park Jogger: A Story of Hope and Possibility*. New York: Scribner, 2004.

Phillips, Helen. "'Rewired Brain' Revives Patient after 19 Years." *New Scientist* (July 3, 2006).

Prohl, J., J. Röther, S. Kluge, G. de Heer, J. Liepert, S. Bodenburg, K. Pawlik, and G. Kreymann. "Prediction of Short-Term and Long-Term Outcomes after Cardiac Arrest: A prospective Multivariate Approach Combining Biochemical, Clinical, Electrophysiological, and Neuropsychological Investigations." *Critical Care Medicine* 35, no. 5 (May 2007): 1230–1237.

Sabom, Michael. *Recollections of Death: A Medical Investigation.* New York: Harper & Row, 1982.

Schumann, John Henning. "The Worst Fortune Tellers: Why Doctors Are So Bad at Predicting How Long Their Patients Will Live." *Slate*, August 18, 2010.

Thomas, Gordon. *Mysteries of the Human Body: Medical Miracles and Unexplained Phenomena of Human Biology.* London: Carlton Books, 2005, pages 4, 10, 13, 35, 40, 43, 50, 53, 60, 61, 64, 67, 71, 10, 115, 137, 139, 143, 149.

Von Hildebrand, Dietrich. *Liturgy and Personality: The Healing Power of Formal Prayer.* Manchester, NH: Sophia Institute Press, 1993.

Interview

Long, Jeffrey, MD, founder of the Near Death Experience Research Foundation, phone interview, July 12, 2007.

3. One Patient, Many Pulses

Ahles, T. A., M. B. Yunus, S.D. Riley, J. M. Bradley, A. T. Masi. "Psychological Factors Associated with Primary Fibromyalgia Syndrome." *Arthritis & Rheumatism* 27, 10 (1984): 1101–1106.

American Diabetes Association. "Diagnosis and Classification of Diabetes Mellitus." *Diabetes Care* 33, Suppl 1 (2010): S62–S69.

———."Standards of Medical Care in Diabetes—2010." *Diabetes Care* 33, Suppl 1 (2010): S11–S61.

American Psychiatric Association. "Diagnostic Criteria for 300.14 Dissociative Identity Disorder." *Diagnostic and Statistical Manual of Mental Disorders*, 4th ed., text revision (DSM-IV-TR) ed., 2000, behavenet.com/capsules/. Retrieved March 14, 2010.

Bennett, E. J., C. C. Tennant, C. Piesse, C. A. Badcock, and J. E. Kellow. "Level of Chronic Life Stress Predicts Clinical Outcome in Irritable Bowel Syndrome." *Gut* 43, no. 2 (1998): 256–261.

Bradley, Margaret M., and Peter J. Lang. "Measuring Emotion, Behavior Feeling, and Physiology." In Richard D. Lane, and Lynn Nadel, *Cognitive Neuroscience of Emotion*. New York: Oxford University Press, 2002.

Burckhardt, C. S., S. R. Clark, and R. M. Bennett. "Fibromyalgia and Quality of Life: A Comparative Analysis." *Journal of Rheumatology* 20, no. 3 (1993): 475–479.

"Burning or Tingling Feet May Be Early Warning of Pre-Diabetes." *University of Michigan Health Minute Update*, www.med.umich.edu/opm/newspage/2005/hmprediabetes.htm, June 28, 2005.

Canataroglu, A., Y. Gumurdulu, A. Erdem, and S. Colakoglu. "Prevalence of Fibromyalgia in Patients with Irritable Bowel Syndrome." *The Turkish Journal of Gastroenteroly* 12, no. 2 (2001): 141144.

Carter, L. E., D. W. McNeil, K. E. Vowles, J. T. Sorrell, C. L. Turk, B. J. Ries, and D. R. Hopko. "Effects of Emotion on Pain Reports, Tolerance and Physiology." *Pain Research & Management*, 7, no. 1 (Spring 2000): 21–30.

"Diabetes." Medline Plus, www.nlm.nih.gov/medlineplus/ency/article/001214.htm, updated October 26, 2010.

Eisenbarth, G. S., K. S. Polonsky, and J. B. Buse. "Type 1 Diabetes Mellitus." In H. M. Kronenberg, S. Melmed, K. S. Polonsky, and P. R. Larsen. *Kronenberg: Williams Textbook of Endocrinology*, 11th ed. Philadelphia, PA: Saunders Elsevier, 2008.

Gross, J. J. "Antecedent-and Response-Focused Emotion Regulation: Divergent Consequences for Experience, Expression, and Physiology." *Journal of Personality and Social Psychology* 74(1), (1998). 224–237.

Kluft, R. P. "Iatrongenic Creation of New Alter Personalities" (PDF). *Dissociation* 2, no. 2 (1989): 83–91, https://scholarsbank.uoregon.edu/dspace/bitstream/1794/1428/1/Diss_2_2_6_OCR.pdf. Retrieved April 21, 2008.

Lipton, Bruce H. *The Biology of Belief: Unleashing the Power of Consciousness, Matter, & Miracles*. Carlsbad, CA: Hay House, 2008.

Loewenstein, Richard J. "DID 101: A Hands-on Clinical Guide to the Stabilization Phase of Dissociative Identity Disorder Treatment." Trauma Disorders Program, Sheppard Pratt Health Systems. *Psychiatric Clinics of North America* 29, no. 1 (2006)305–332, xii.

McGowan, P. O., et al. "Epigenetic Regulation of the Glucocorticoid Receptor in Human Brain Associates with Childhood Abuse." *Nature Neuroscience* 12 (2009): 342–348. Published online February 22, 2009.

Schwarz, E., and B. D. Perry. The Post-Traumatic Response in Children and Adolescents. *Psychiatric Clinics of North America* 17, no. 2 (1994): 311–326.

Siegel, Marc. "Struggling with Identities in the United States of Tara." *LA Times Health*, February 23, 2009.

Warren S., S. Greenhill, and K. G. Warren. "Emotional Stress and the Development of Multiple Sclerosis: Case-Control Evidence of a Relationship." *Journal of Chronic Diseases* 35, no. 11 (1982): 821–831.

Zautra, A. J., M. H. Burleson, K. S. Matt, S. Roth, L. Burrows. "Interpersonal Stress, Depression, and Disease Activity in Rheumatoid Arthritis and Osteoarthritis Patients." *Health Psychology* 13, no. 2 (1994): 139–148.

Interviews

Kluft, Richard, MD, PhD, clinical professor of psychiatry and Temple University School of Medicine, former president of the International Society for the Study of Trauma and Dissociation, February 10, 2009.

Loewenstein, Richard, MD, senior psychiatrist and founder and medical director of the Trauma Disorders Program at Sheppard Pratt Health Systems, February 12, 2009.

Shatkin, Jess, MD, MPH, director of education and training, NYU Child Study Center, February 12, 2009.

4. Inner Pulse Rising

Bader, Garin. *Psycho-Cybernetics*. New York: Pocket, THUS edition, August 15th, 1989.

Bailey-Lloyd, C./Lady Camelot. "The Incredible Human Psyche." *Holistic Junction*, psychology.articlesarchive.net/the-incredible-human-psyche1.html, accessed July 22, 2007.

Behm, D. G., K. Power, and E. Drinkwater. "Muscle Activation Is Enhanced with Multi- and Uni-Articular Bilateral versus Unilateral Contractions." *Canadian Journal of Applied Physiology* 28, no. 1 (2002): 38–52.

Behm, D. G., PhD, J. Whittle, BSc, D. Button, BKin, and K. Power, BKin. "Intermuscle Differences in Activation." *Muscle & Nerve* 25 (2002): 236–243.

George, Jane. "Polar Bear No Match for Fearsome Mother in Ivujivik." *Nunatsiaq News*, February 17, 2006.

Gonzales, Laurence. *Deep Survival: Who Lives, Who Dies, and Why.* New York: W. W. Norton, 2004.

Goodstein, Laurie, and William Glaberson. "The Well-Marked Roads to Homicidal Rage." *New York Times*, April 10, 2010.

Hopkins, Will. "Summary: Feats of Extreme Strength and Power." Sportscience, www.mail-archive.com/sportscience@yahoogroups.com/msg00157.html, accessed July 16, 2007.

"Hypnosis." Acupuncture and Therapeutic Bodywork. Total Care Medical Center, Palo Alto, CA, www.totalcare.org/hypnosis.htm, accessed July 15, 2007.

Ikai, Michio, and Arthur H. Steinhaus. "Some Factors Modifying the Expression of Human Strength." *Journal of Applied Physiology* 16 (1961): 157–163.

"Inclusion Body Myositis—Treatment Information, Diagnosis, Symptoms." Johns Hopkins Medicine, www.hopkinsmedicine.org/myositis/myositis/ibm.html, accessed June 8, 2009.

"Matt Furey Uncensored: Lift a Car with One Arm," www.mattfurey.com/testimonials.html, accessed July 18, 2010.

McArdle, William D., Frank I. Katch, and Victor L. Katch. *Exercise Physiology: Nutrition, Energy, and Human Performance*, 7th ed. Piladelphia, PA: Lippincott Williams & Wilkins, 2009.

Memmott, Mark. "Arizona Man Lifts Car off Injured Teen." USA Today, blogs.usatoday.com/ondeadline/2006/07/arizona_man_lif.html, posted July 28, 2006, at 4 p.m.

Moore, Nicole N., Maj. USAF, MC, and John Michael Bostwick, MD. "Ketamine Dependence in Anesthesia Providers." *Psychosomatics* 40 (August 1999): 356–359.

Orne, M. T. "Hypnosis, Motivation, and Compliance." *American Journal of Psychiatry* 122 (1966): 721–726.

Rashbaum, William K. "Police Say Ex-Employee Shoots Lawyer." *New York Times*, September 22, 2000.

Roby, Russell, MD, JD. "Chronic Fatigue Syndrome." Roby Institute, Advanced Treatments for Healthy Living, www.onlineallergycenter.com/treatments/chronic_fatigue_syndrome_cfs.htm, accessed July 16, 2007.

Siegel, Marc. "The Emotions of Attack." *San Francisco Chronicle*, December 31, 2007.

Sternberg, Eliezer J. *Are You a Machine? The Brain, the Mind, and What It Means to Be Human*: Amherst, NY: Humanity Books, 2007.

"The Excited Delirium Syndrome." In *Custody Deaths: Excited Delirium: Operations & Tactics* at Officer.com, www.officer.com/web/online/Opertions-and-Tactics/In-Custody-Deaths--Excited-Delirium-Syndrome, accessed July 16, 2007.

"Transformation Works—Hypnosis and Self-Hypnosis for Mind and Body Healing," Healing with Hypnosis, www.tranceformation.com/trance .mv?ARTID=hypfaq, accessed July 22, 2007.

"True Story of Superhuman Strength on 9-11: Eyewitness Account from Inside WTC 1," America Stands Tall, americastandstall.org/stories/sabrina .html, accessed July 18, 2007.

Waterworth, S. P., and G. R. H. Sandercock. "The Reliability of a New Method of Measuring Stiffness of the Human Hamstrings Muscles." *Journal of Sports Sciences* 19, no.1 (2001): 7.

5. Radar to Die

"Aberfan Landslide Disaster: October 22, 1966." WalesOnline, www .walesonline.co.uk/news/welsh-history/2010/09/13/western-mail-22nd-october-1966-aberfan-91466-27258419/, accessed July 23, 2007.

Bierman, Dick J., and H. Steven Scholte. "Anomalous Anticipatory Brain Activation Preceding Exposure of Emotional and Neutral Pictures." *Journal of Parapsychology* 11 (2), (2002) 163–180.

Bierman, D. J., and D. I. Radin. "Anomalous Anticipatory Response on Randomized Future Conditions." *Perceptual and Motor Skills* 84 (1997): 689–690.

Dosa, David M., MD, MPH. "A Day in the Life of Oscar the Cat." Perspective. *New England Journal of Medicine* 357; 4 (July 26, 2007): 328–329.

Dosa, David. *Making Rounds with Oscar: The Extraordinary Gift of an Ordinary Cat*, 1st ed. New York: Hyperion, 2010.

Guiley, Rosemary Ellen. *Harper's Encyclopedia of Mystical and Paranormal Experience*. New York: HarperCollins, 1991.

Hevesi, Dennis. "Rabbi Zev Segal, Orthodox Leader Who Took Interfaith Approach to Social Issues, Dies at 91." *New York Times*, March 9, 2008.

Hildrum, B., et al. "Effect of Anxiety and Depression on Blood Pressure: 11-Year Longitudinal Population Study." *British Journal of Psychiatry* 193 (2008): 108.

"Premonition"The Mystica, www.themystica.com/mystica/articles/p/premonition .html, accessed July 23, 2007.

Radin, Dean. *Entangled Minds: Extrasensory Experiences in a Quantum Reality*. New York: Paraview Pocket Books, 2006.

———. DeanRadin, www.deanradin.com/NewWeb/bio.html, accessed July 29, 2007.

Robertson, Morgan, and Ian Stevenson, MD. *The Wreck of the Titanic: The Paranormal Experiences Connected with the Sinking of the Titanic*. Cutchogue, NY: Buccaneer Books, 1991.

Sheps, S. G., ed. *Mayo Clinic 5 Steps to Controlling High Blood Pressure*. Rochester, MN: Mayo Foundation for Medical Education and Research, 2008.

Spence, Lewis. *An Encyclopedia of Occultism*. New York: Carol Publishing Group Edition, 1996.

Wei, T. M., et al. "Anxiety Symptoms in Patients with Hypertension: A Community-Based Study. *International Journal of Psychiatry in Medicine* 36 (2006): 315.

Interview

David Dosa, MD, February 10, 2010.

6. Dancing in the Dark

Ballen, William. "Freud's Views and the Contemporary Application of Hypnosis: Enhancing Therapy within a Psychoanalytic Framework." *Journal of Contemporary Psychotherapy* 27, no. 3 (1997): 201–214, 6.

Bourgnignon, Erika, ed. *Religion, Altered States of Consciousness and Social Change*. Columbia: Ohio University Press, 1973.

Braverman, Lewis E., and Robert D. Utiger, eds. Werner & Ingbar's *The Thyroid: A Fundamental & Clinical Text*, 9th ed. Philadelphia, PA: Lippincott Williams & Wilkins, 2005.

Freud, Sigmund, and Joseph Breuer. *Studies on Hysteria (1893–1895)*. New York: Basic Books Classics 2000, originally published London: Hogarth Press, 1895.

Harrington, Anne. "Possession, Exorcism, and Their First Skeptics." In *The Cure Within: A History of Mind-Body Medicine*. New York: W. W. Norton, 2008.

Hogarth, Robin M. *Educating Intuition*. Chicago, IL: University of Chicago Press, 2001.

Lee, Catherine See-Ning, and Burton Hutto. "Recognizing Thyrotoxicosis in a Patient with Bipolar Mania: A Case Report." *Annals of General Psychiatry* 7:3 (2008).

Nath, Jisu, and Rajesh Sagar. "Late-Onset Bipolar Disorder due to Hyperthyroidism." *Acta Psychiatrica Scandinavica* 104, no. 1 (July 2001): 72–75.

"NIH Launches Undiagnosed Diseases Program." *NIH News*, May 19, 2008, www.nih.gov.

Norman, James. "Thyroiditis." EndocrineWeb, www.endocrineweb.com/conditions/thyroid/thyroiditis, published March 29, 2009, updated October 13, 2010.

Stowell, Charles P., MD, and John W. Barnhill, MD. "Acute Mania in the Setting of Severe Hypothyroidism." *Psychosomatics* 46 (June 2005): 259–261.

7. Infection of Body, Infection of Spirit

"Battle of the Bugs: Fighting Antibiotic Resistance" FDA www.fda.gov/Drugs/ResourcesForYou/Consumers/ucm143568.htm, accessed January 10, 2010.

Brown, Donna Quinton, RN. "Electrocardiography Wires: A Potential Source of Infection." *AACN News* 23, no. 9 September 2006): 12–15.

"CDC Estimates 94,000 Invasive Drug-Resistant Staph Infections Occurred in the U.S. in 2005." CDC, www.cdc.gov/media/pressrel/2007/r071016.htm?s_cid=mediarel_r071016, October 16, 2007.

Cohen, Sheldon, David A. J. Tyrrell, and Andrew P. Smith. "Negative Life Events, Perceived Stress, Negative Affect, and Susceptibility to the Common Cold." *Journal of Personality and Social Psychology* 64, no. 1 (1993): 131–140.

Cohen, S., D. A. Tyrrell , and A. P. Smith. "Psychological Stress and Susceptibility to the Common Cold." *N Engl J Med* 325, no. 9 (August 1991): 606–612.

Cristomo, M. I., H. Westh, A. Tomasz, M. Chung, D. C. Olivera, and H. de Lencastre. "The Evolution of Methicillin Resistance in Staphylococcus." *Proceedings of the National Academy of Sciences of the United States of America* 99 (2002): 7687–7692.

"Deaths involving MRSA and Clostridium Difficile by Communal Establishment: England and Wales, 2001–06." *Health Statistics Quarterly* 38, *Office for National Statistics* (Summer 2008).

Gottlieb, Scott. "Attack of the Superbugs." Opinion. *Wall Street Journal*, October 30, 2007.

Humphries, Jodie. "The Real State of Hospital Cleanliness." *EHM, Executive Healthcare* no. 8, "Infection Control" (July 2009).

Klevens, R. Monina, DDS, MPH, Melissa A. Morrison, MPH, Joelle Nadle, MPH, Susan Petit, MPH, Ken Gershman, MD, MPH, Susan Ray, MD, et al., for the Active Bacterial Core Surveillance (ABCs) MRSA Investigators. "Invasive Methicillin-Resistant Staphylococcus Aureus Infections in the United States." *Journal of the American Medical Association* 298 (2007): 1763–1771.

Lankford, M., S. Collins, L. Youngberg, D. Rooney, J. Warren, and G. Noskin. "Assessment of Materials Commonly Utilized in Healthcare: Implications for Bacterial Survival and Transmission." *American Journal of Infection Control* 34 , no. 5 (June 2006): 258–263.

McCaughey, Betsy. "Hospital Scrubs Are a Germy Deadly Mess." *Wall Street Journal*, Opinion, January 8, 2009.

———. "Why Aren't Hospitals Cleaner?" *US News and World Report*, July 16, 2007.

"Medical Fabrics: A Reservoir of Pathogenic Bacterium?" *Infection Control Today*, December 31, 2008, www.infectioncontroltoday.com/articles/2008/ 12/medical-fabrics-a-reservoir-of-pathogenic-bacteri.aspx.

Milam, M. W., M. Hall, T. Pringle, and K. Buchanan. "Bacterial Contamination of Fabric Stethoscope Covers: The Velveteen Rabbit of Health Care?" *Infection Control and Hospital Epidemiology* 22, no. 10 (October 2001): 653–655.

Montero, Douglas, and Chuck Bennett. "Brave to the End." *New York Post*, October 31, 2007.

Neely, A. N., and M. P. Maley. "Survival of Enterococci and Staphylococci on Hospital Fabrics and Plastic." *Journal of Clinical Microbiology* 38, no. 2 (February 2000): 724–726.

Pilonetto, M., E. A. R Rosa, P. R. S. Brofman, D. Baggio, F. Calvário, C. Schelp, A. Nascimento, and I. Messias-Reason. "Hospital Gowns as a Vehicle for Bacterial Dissemination in an Intensive Care Unit." *Brazilian Journal of Infectious Diseases* 8, no. 3 (June 2004).

"Regaining Control of MRSA." Delmarva Foundation, www.positivedeviance .org/pdf/publications/Delmarva.pdf, accessed January 10, 2009.

Schaubroeck, J., and J. R. Jones. "Individual Differences in Utilizing Control to Cope with Job Demands: Effects on Susceptibility to Infectious Disease." *Journal of Applied Psychology* 86, no. 2 (2001): 265–278.

Siegel, Marc. "Rx for the 'Superbug.'" *NY Post*, Opinion, October 31, 2007.

Sullivan, C. J., Yoav Gonen, and Andy Geller. "Superbug Strikes in City, Brooklyn Schoolboy, 12, Dies of Infection." *New York Post*, October 26, 2007.

Wilson, J., H. Loveday, P. Hoffman, and R. Pratt. *Uniform: An Evidence Review of the Microbiological Significance of Uniforms and Uniform Policy in the Prevention and Control of Healthcare-Associated Infections*. Report to the Department of Health (England). *Journal of Hospital Infection* 66, no. 4 (2007): 301–307.

8. Never Say Die

Basinger, David, and Richard Basinger, eds. *Predestination and Free Will*. Downers Grove, IL: IVP Academic, 1986.

Beilby, James K., and Paul R. Eddy, eds. *Divine Foreknowledge: Four Views*. Downers Grove, IL: IVP Academic, 2001.

Block, S. D., and J. A. Billings. "Patient Requests to Hasten Death. Evaluation and Management in Terminal Care." *Archives of Internal Medicine* 154 (1994): 2039–2047.

Block, Susan D., MD. "Assessing and Managing Depression in the Terminally Ill Patient." *Focus, Psychiatry* 3 (2005): 310–319.

Breitbart, W., E. Bruera, H. Chochinov, and M. Lynch. "Neuropsychiatric Syndromes and Psychological Symptoms in Patients with Advanced Cancer." *Journal of Pain Symptom Management* 10 (1995):131–141.

Cloughesy, T. F., M. D. Prados, P. Y. Wen, T. Mikkelsen, L. E. Abrey, D. Schiff, W. K. Yung, Z. Maoxia, I. Dimery, and H. S. Friedman. "A Phase II, Randomized, Non-Comparative Clinical Trial of the Effect of Bevacizumab (BV) Alone or in Combination with Irinotecan (CPT) on 6-Month Progression Free Survival (PFS6) in Recurrent, Treatment-Refractory Glioblastoma (GBM)." 2008 ASCO Annual Meeting Proceedings (Post-Meeting Edition). *Journal of Clinical Oncology* 26, no. 15S (May 20 Supplement, 2008): 2010b.

Coyne, James C., Thomas F. Pajak, Jonathan Harris, Andre Konski, Benjamin Movsas, Kian Ang, and Deborah Watkins Bruner. "Emotional Well-Being Does Not Predict Survival in Head and Neck Cancer Patients: A Radiation Therapy Oncology Group Study." *Cancer*, Published Online (October 2007).

Groopman, Jerome E. *The Anatomy of Hope*. New York: Random House Trade Paperbacks, 2005.

Kadden, Barbara, and Bruce Kadden. *Teaching Mitzvot: Concepts, Values, and Activities.* Denver, CO: A.R.E. Publishing, 2003.

Levy, Ze'ev, and Yudit Kornberg Greenberg. *From Spinoza to Lévinas: Hermeneutical, Ethical, and Political Issues in Modern and Contemporary Jewish Philosophy.* New York: Peter Lang, 2009.

Nuland, Sherwin B. *Maimonides.* New York: Schocken, 1st reprint edition, 2008.

Oppenheimer, Mark. "The Turning of an Atheist." *New York Times Magazine,* November 4, 2007.

Sampson, J. H., A. B. Heimberger, G. E. Archer, K. D. Aldape, A. H. Friedman, H. S. Friedman, M.R. Gilbert, J. E. Herndon 2nd, R. E. McLendon, D. A. Mitchell, D. A. Reardon, Sawaya, R. J. Schmittling, W. Shi , J. J. Vredenburgh, and D. D. Bigner. "Immunologic Escape after Prolonged Progression-Free Survival with Epidermal Growth Factor Receptor Variant III Peptide Vaccination in Patients with Newly Diagnosed Glioblastoma." *Journal of Clinical Oncology* 28, no. 31 (November 1, 2010): 4722–4729. E-published October 4, 2010.

Segal, Rabbi Arthur. "Talmud Yerushalmi Bikkurim: Aging with God: Counting the Omer." Zimbio, Judaism, www.zimbio.com/Judaism/articles/75/RABBI+ARTHUR+SEGAL+TALMUD+YERUSHALMI+BIKKURIM, accessed May 2, 2008.

Sheikh, Rafiq A., MB, MD, MRCP (UK), FACP, FACG, Shagufta Yasmeen, MD, MRCOG (London), and Thomas Prindiville, MD: "Toxic Megacolon: A Review," *JK- Practitioner, International Journal of Current Medical Science & Practice* 10, no. 3 (July–September 2003): 176–178.

Spiegel, D., J. Bloom, H. Kraemer, and E. Gottheil. "Effect of Psychosocial Treatment on Survival of Patients with Metastatic Breast Cancer." *Lancet* 2 (1989): 888–891.

Sproul, R. C. *Chosen by God.* Carol Stream, IL: Tyndale House, 1994.

Twersky, Isadore, ed. *A Maimonides Reader,* 1st ed. Springfield, NJ: Behrman House, 1972.

Interviews

Gruber, Michael, MD, professor of neuro-oncology at NYU Langone Medical Center, April 11, 2008.

Pachter, Leon, MD, chief of surgery, NYU Langone Medical Center, March 23, 2007.

9. Radar to Live

Berg, Yehuda. *Kabbalah: The Power to Change Everything*. Los Angeles, CA: Kabbalah Publishing, 2009.

"CT Screening of Former, Current Smokers Reduces Lung Cancer Deaths, Study Finds." *ScienceDaily*, November 5, 2010.

Haftarah for Eikev, Isaiah 49:14–51:3, The Jewish Theological Seminary, www.jtsa.edu/PreBuilt/ParashahArchives/jpstext/ekev_haft.shtml, accessed June 9, 2008.

Horton, Robert Forman. "The Beginning of Wisdom." In *The Book of Proverbs*. Whitefish, MT: Kessinger Publishing, 2010.

Huss, Boaz, Marco Pasi, and Kocku Von Stuckrad, eds. *Kabbalah and Modernity: Interpretations, Transformations, Adaptations*. Leiden, The Netherlands: Aries Book Series, BRILL, 2010.

Samuel, Gabriella. *The Kabbalah Handbook: A Concise Encyclopedia of Terms and Concepts in Jewish Mysticism*. New York: Tarcher, 2007.

Siegel, Marc. "Common Sense Medicine." *National Review Online*, www.nationalreview.com/articles/252722/common-sense-medicine-nro-editors.

Sloan, Richard P. *Blind Faith: The Unholy Alliance of Religion and Medicine*. New York: St. Martin's Griffin, 1st reprint edition, 2008.

Williams, William Carlos. *The Doctor Stories*, 1st ed. New York: New Directions, 1984.

10. The Black Swan

Beck-Peccoz, P., and L. Persani. "Premature Ovarian Failure." *Orphanet Journal of Rare Diseases* 1 (2006): 9.

Blumenfeld, Z., S. Halachmi, B. A. Peretz, Z. Shmuel, D. Golan, A. Makler, and J. M. Brandes. "Premature Ovarian Failure—The Prognostic Application of Autoimmunity on Conception after Ovulation Induction." *Fertility and Sterility* 59, no. 4 (1993): 750–755.

Clarke, David D., MD. *They Can't Find Anything Wrong! 7 Keys to Understanding, Treating, and Healing Stress Illness*, 1st ed. Boulder, CO: Sentient Publications, 2007).

Doody, K. M., and B. R. Carr. "Amenorrhea." *Obstetrics & Gynecology Clinics of North America* 17 (1990): 361–387.

Groopman, Jerome E. *How Doctors Think*. Boston, MA: Houghton Mifflin, 2007.

Kalantaridou, S. N., and L. M. Nelson. "Premature Ovarian Failure Is Not Premature Menopause." *Annals of New York Academy of Sciences* 900 (2000): 393–402.

Mann, Thomas. *The Black Swan*, 1st ed. New York: Alfred A. Knopf, 1954.

Speroff, L., R. H. Glass, and N. G. Kase, eds. *Menstrual Disorders in Gynecologic Endocrinology and Infertility*, 6th ed. Philadelphia, PA: Lippincott Williams & Wilkins, 1999.

Tulandi, T., and R. Kinch. "A Prospective Study of Women with Premature Ovarian Failure." *Fertility Sterility* 40 (1983): 279.

Interview

David D. Clarke, MD, clinical assistant professor of gastroenterology emeritus and senior scholar at the Center for Ethics at Oregon Health and Science University, December 10, 2007.

11. The Truth about Psychic Healing

Benor, Daniel J. "Controlled Studies." In *Spiritual Healing: Scientific Validation of a Healing Revolution*. Bellmawr, NJ: Wholistic Healing, 2006.

Bro, Harmon Hartzell. *Edgar Cayce: A Seer out of Season*. London: Aquarian Press, 1990.

Cerminara, Dr. Gina. "The Medical Clairvoyance of Edgar Cayce." In *Many Mansions, The Edgar Cayce Story on Reincarnation*. New York: Signet Book, 1950, reissued 1990.

Edwards, Harry. *A Guide to Spirit Healing*. Bel Air, CA: Hesperides Press, 2008.

Fuina, Anthony M. "Anthony Fuina's Testimony of God's Miraculous Healing Grace." Signs, Wonders, and Miracles, www.christian-miracles.com/anthonyfuinasmiracle.htm, accessed March 9, 2009.

———. "Padre Pio, My Greatest Miracle." January 7, 2001, www.messenger ofpadrepio.com/docs/MyGreatestMiracle.pdf, accessed March 9, 2009.

Licauco, Jaime T. *Born to Heal, the Amazing Story of Spiritual Healer Rev. Alex Orbito*. Published by the author, 1986.

"Maria Regina R.C. Church Held Its Celebratory Mass and Dedication of the Padre Pio of Pietrelcina, December 10, 2006," LongIslandNews, www .massapequanews.com/education/mariaregina.html, accessed March 9, 2009.

Miller, Paul. *Born to Heal: A Biography of Harry Edwards, the Spirit Healer*. London: Corgi Childrens, New Ed edition, 1972.

Mosconi, Angela. "Miraculous Cure Recalled." *New York Daily News*, March 31, 2002.

Sawhney, Clifford. "Spiritual Healing—Psychic Surgery Uncovered" (about Alex Orbito). *Life Positive*, February 2001.

Interview

Anthony Fuina, long-time parishioner of St. William the Abbot Parish in Seaford, New York, conducted March 13, 2009.

12. The Strongest Inner Pulse

Blaine, David. *Mysterious Stranger*. New York: Villard Books, a Division of Random House, 2002.

———. See David Blaine Web site, davidblaine.com/, accessed February 10, 2009 .

———. Dr. Posner letter from David Blaine Web site, davidblaine.flux .com/News/Letter-to-Dr-Ruden/0C4DBFFFF0195BB31001600A7EDE5, accessed February 10, 2009.

Korbonits, M., D. Blaine, M. Elia, and J. Powell-Tuck. "Refeeding David Blaine: Studies after a 44-Day Fast." *New England Journal of Medicine* 353, no. 21 (November 24, 2005): 2306–2307.

"Longest Breath Holding-World Record Set by David Blaine." Worldrecordsacademy.org, www.worldrecordsacademy.org/stunts/longest_breathholding_world_record_set_by_David_Blaine_80235.htm, accessed February 12, 2009.

Silverman, Kenneth. *Houdini!!! The Career of Ehrich Weiss, American Self-Liberator, Europe's Eclipsing Sensation, World's Handcuff King & Prison Breaker*. New York: HarperCollins, 1996.

Tierney, John. "David Blaine Sets Breath-Holding Record." *New York Times*, April 30, 2008.

Woog, Adam. *Harry Houdini*. Farmington Hills, MI: Lucent Books, 1995.

Interview

David Blaine, magician and endurance artist, conducted at his offices, February 10, 2009.

13. Who Dies? Who Lives?

Block, Keith I. "Antineoplastons and the Challenges of Research in Integrative Care." *Integrative Cancer Therapies* 3, no. 1 (2004): 3–4.

Burzynski, S. R., T. J. Janicki, R. A. Weaver, and B. Burzynski. "Targeted Therapy with Antineoplastons A10 and AS2-1 of High-Grade, Recurrent, and Progressive Brainstem Glioma." *Integrative Cancer Therapies* 5, no. 1 (2006): 40–47.

Cao, Yihai, and Robert Langer. "A Review of Judah Folkman's Remarkable Achievements in Biomedicine." *Proceedings of the National Academy of Sciences, United States of America* 105, no. 36 (September 9, 2008): 13203–13205.2

Chekhov, Anton. *Ward Six and Other Stories*. Meridian Classics. New York: Plume, 1965.

Cohen, M. A., and P. McGrady Jr. "Emanuel Revici, MD, Age 101, Medical Innovator." *Townsend Letter for Doctors & Patients* 177 (April 1998): 30–31.

Cohen, M. "Emanuel Revici, MD: Innovator in Nontoxic Cancer Chemotherapy 1896–1997." *Journal of Alternative & Complementary Medicine* 4, no. 2 (Summer 1998): 140–145.

El-Serag, H. B., J. A. Marrero, L. Rudolph, and K. R. Reddy. "Diagnosis and Treatment of Hepatocellular Carcinoma." *Gastroenterology* 134, no. 6 (May 2008): 1752–1763.

Gellert, G. A., R. M. Maxwell, and B. S. Siegel. "Survival of Breast Cancer Patients Receiving Adjunctive Psychosocial Support Therapy: A 10-Year Follow-up Study." *Journal of Clinical Oncology* 11, no. 1 (January 1993): 66–69.

Harrington, Anne. "The Body That Speaks." In *The Cure Within: A History of Mind-Body Medicine*. New York: W.W. Norton, 2008.

Hepatocellular Carcinoma—Screening, Diagnosis, and Management. Natcher Conference Center, National Institutes of Health, Bethesda, Maryland, April 1–3, 2004, www3.niddk.nih.gov/fund/other/hepato_carc/liver_cancer.pdf, accessed March 22, 2009.

Hoshida, Yujin, MD, PhD, Augusto Villanueva, MD, Masahiro Kobayashi, MD, et al. "Gene Expression in Fixed Tissues and Outcome in Hepatocellular Carcinoma." *N Engl J Med* 359 (2008): 1995–2004.

Lyall, D., M. Schwartz, F. P. Herter, et al. "Treatment of Cancer by the Method of Revici." *Journal of the American Medical Association*, 194 (1965): 279–280.

Pawlotsky, J. M., F. Roudot-Thoraval, C. Pellet, P. Aumont, F. Darthuy, J. Remire, J. Duval, and D. Dhumeaux. "Influence of Hepatitis C Virus (HCV) Genotypes on HCV Recombinant Immunoblot Assay Patterns." *Journal of Clinical Microbiology* 33, no. 5 (May 1995): 1357–1359.

"The Practice of Dr. Emanuel Revici." See Revici Medical Research, www.revicimedical.com, accessed April 2, 2009.

"Revici's Guided Chemotherapy." American Cancer Society, www.cancer.org/Treatment/TreatmentsandSideEffects/ComplementaryandAlternativeMedicine/PharmacologicalandBiologicalTreatment/revicis-guided-chemotherapy, accessed March 30, 2009.

"Revici Guided Chemotherapy Detailed Scientific Review." MD Anderson Cancer Center, www.mdanderson.org/education-and-research/resources-for-professionals/clinical-tools-and-resources/cimer/therapies/nonplant-biologic-organic-pharmacologic-therapies/revici-scientific.html, accessed April 6, 2009.

Siegel, Bernie S., MD. *Love, Medicine, & Miracles.* New York: Harper & Row, c. 1986; other printing edition, 1986.

Sontag, Susan. *Illness as Metaphor*, 1st ed. New York: Farrar, Straus and Giroux, 1978.

"Unproven Methods of Cancer Management: Revici Method." American Cancer Society, *CA: A Cancer Journal for Clinicians* 39 (1989): 119122.

Vickers, A. "Alternative Cancer Cures: 'Unproven' or 'Disproven'?" *CA* 54, no. 2 (2004): 110–118.

14. Considering the Alternative

Adair, F. E., R. C. Mellors, J. H. Farrow, H. Q. Woodard, G. C. Escher, and J. A. Urban. "The Use of Estrogens and Androgens in Advanced Mammary Cancer: Clinical and Laboratory Study of One Hundred and Five Female Patients." *Journal of the American Medical Association* 140, no. 15 (August 13, 1949): 1193–1200.

Altman, Shem. "Persistent Patients Find Answers." *Families on-the-go Magazine*, January–February 2007, www.familiesonthego.org/health/health-0032.htm, accessed May 13, 2009.

Barnes, P., E. Powell-Griner, K. McFann, and R. Nahin. *CDC Advance Data Report #343. Complementary and Alternative Medicine Use among Adults: United States, 2002.* May 27, 2004.

Bausell, R. Barker, PhD. *Snake Oil Science: The Truth about Complementary and Alternative Medicine*, 1st ed. New York: Oxford University Press, 2007.

Cutly, M., and M. Schlemenson. "Treatment of Advanced Mammary Cancer with Testosterone." *Journal of the American Medical Association* 138, no. 3 (September 18, 1948): 187–190.

Cutshall, Susanne M., Laura L. Fenske, Ryan F. Kelly, Brent R. Phillips, Thoralf M. Sundt, and Brent A. Bauer. "Creation of a Healing Enhancement Program at an Academic Medical Center." *Complementary Therapies in Clinical Practice* 13, no. 4 (November 2007): 217–223.

Ernster, V. L., R. Ballard-Barbash, and W. E. Barlow, et al. "Detection of Ductal Carcinoma in Situ in Women Undergoing Screening Mammography." *Journal of the National Cancer Institute* 94, no. 20 (October 2002): 1546–1554.

Fels, Eric, MD. "Treatment of Breast Cancer with Testosterone Propionate." *Journal of Clinical Endocrinology* 4, no. 3 (1944): 121–125.

Gill, Lisa. "More Hospitals Offer Alternative Therapies for Mind, Body, Spirit." *USA Today*, September 15, 2008.

Kilham, Chris. "Herbs to Boost Health and Profits." *Science Now, Functional Ingredients* (April 2010).

Marinac, Jacqueline S., PharmD, Colleen L. Buchinger, MD, Lincoln A. Godfrey, DO, James M. Wooten, PharmD, Chao Sun, MD, MPH, and Sandra K. Willsie, DO. "Herbal Products and Dietary Supplements: A Survey of Use, Attitudes, and Knowledge among Older Adults." *Journal of the American Osteopathic Association* 107, no. 1 (January 2007): 13–23.

Svane, Gunilla. "Ductal Carcinoma in Situ (DCIS): Incidence, Prognosis, and Diagnostic Aspects of Mammography, Galactography, and Needle Biopsies." In *Research and Development in Breast Ultrasound*, ed. E. Ueno, Shiina, T., Kubota, M., and Sawai, K. New York: Springer, 2005, 114–118.

Interview

Shem Altman, MD, chemical pathologist in Paradise Valley, Arizona, interview on May 12, 2009.

15. Miracles and the Inner Pulse

Aquinas, Thomas. *Summa Contra Gentiles: Book One: God*. Notre Dame, IN: University of Notre Dame Press, 1991.

Augustine of Hippo. *The City of God against the Pagans*. Translation by R. W. Dyson. New York: Cambridge University Press, 1998.

Barrett, Cyril. *Wittgenstein on Ethics and Religious Belief*. Hoboken, NJ: Blackwell, 1991.

"David Hume." *Stanford Encyclopedia of Philosophy*, Center for the Study of Language and Information, Stanford University, Stanford, CA: first published February 26, 2001; substantive revision May 15, 2009, plato .stanford.edu/entries/hume/, accessed September 13, 2009.

Dein, Simon. "The Power of Words: Healing Narratives among Lubavitcher Hasidim." *Medical Anthropology Quarterly* 16, no. 1: (March 2002) 41–63.

Fogelin, Robert J. *A Defense of Hume on Miracles*. Princeton, NJ: Princeton University Press, 2003.

Holland, R. F. "The Miraculous." *American Philosophical Quarterly* 2 (1965): 43–51.

Hume, David. *Enquiries concerning Human Understanding*. Edited by L. A. Selby-Bigge, 3rd ed. Oxford, UK: Oxford University Press, 1975.

Jacobson, Simon. *Toward a Meaningful Life: The Wisdom of the Rebbe Menachem Mendel Schneerson*. New York: HarperCollins, 2010.

Monk, Ray. *Ludwig Wittgenstein: The Duty of Genius*. New York: Penguin, 2001.

Radcliffe, Elizabeth S. *A Companion to Hume*. Oxford, UK: Blackwell, 2007.

Maimonides. "Jewish Healing." In *Rambam's Sefer HaMadda (The Book of Knowledge)*. Jewish Healing: Religion and Spirituality Training Through Torah and Kabbalah; See www.jewishhealing.com/rambamchap4.html, accessed July 22, 2009.

Serruys, P. W., M. J. Kutryk, and A. T. Ong. "Coronary-Artery Stents." *New England Journal of Medicine* 354, no. 5 (2006): 483–495.

"St. Thomas Aquinas on Eucharistic Miracles." *Summa Theologica, Part III*. Question 76: "Of the Way in Which Christ Is in This Sacrament," Article 8, www.marys-touch.com/truth/aquinas.htm, accessed January 10, 2010.

"Three Natural Miracles." Judaism, Torah, and Jewish Info – Chabad – Lubavitch, www.chabad.org/parshah/article_cdo/aid/46079/jewish/Three-Natural-Miracles.htm, accessed January 15, 2010.

Touger, Eliyahu. "The Quality of Mercy," Sichos in English. In *To Know and to Care: An Anthology of Chassidic Stories about the Lubavitcher Rebbe Shlita, Rabbi Menachem M. Schneerson*, Brooklyn, NY, Sichos in English, vol. 1.

Yanofsky, Charles S., MD. "The Physician's Oath and Prayer of Maimonides." Translated by Harry Friedenwald. *Bulletin of the Johns Hopkins Hospital* 28 (1917): 260–261, A Catalogue of Physician's Oaths, www.pneuro .com/publications/oaths/#The Physician's Oath and Prayer of Maimonides, accessed July 15, 2009.

Afterword: All in Good Time

Jung, C. G. *Synchronicity, An Acausal Connecting Principle.* Princeton, NJ, Bollingen, 1st Princeton/Bollingen paperback edition, 1973.

Interview

Pachter, Leon, MD, chief of surgery, NYU Langone Medical Center, August 10, 2008.

Recommended Reading

Bausell, R. Barker. *Snake Oil Science: The Truth about Complementary and Alternative Medicine*. New York: Oxford University Press, 2007.

Benor, Daniel J. *Spiritual Healing: Scientific Validation of a Healing Revolution*. Bellmawr, NJ: Wholistic Healing, 2006.

Berg, Yehuda. *Kabbalah: The Power to Change Everything*. Los Angeles: Kabbalah Publishing, 2009.

Blaine, David. *Mysterious Stranger*. New York: Villard Books, a Division of Random House, 2002.

Chekhov, Anton. *Ward Six and Other Stories, Meridian Classics*. New York: Plume, 1965.

Chopra, Deepak. *The Book of Secrets: Unlocking the Hidden Dimensions of Your Life*. New York: Three Rivers Press, 2005.

D'Souza, Dinesh. *Life after Death: The Evidence*. Washington, DC: Regnery Press, 2009.

Dosa, David. *Making Rounds with Oscar: The Extraordinary Gift of an Ordinary Cat*. New York: Hyperion, 2010.

Duffin, Jacalyn. *Medical Miracles: Doctors, Saints, and Healing in the Modern World*. New York: Oxford University Press, 2008.

Frankl, Viktor E. *Man's Search for Meaning*. Cutchogue, NY: Buccaneer Books, 1993.

Freud, Sigmund. *The Uncanny*. New York: Penguin Classics, 2003.

Freud, Sigmund, and Breuer, Joseph. *Studies on Hysteria (1893–1895)*. New York: Basic Books Classics, 2000.

Groopman, Jerome E. *How Doctors Think*. New York: Houghton Mifflin Co., 2007.

———. *The Anatomy of Hope*. New York: Random House Trade Paperbacks, 2005.

Jacobson, Simon. *Toward a Meaningful Life: The Wisdom of the Rebbe Menachem Mendel Schneerson*. New York: HarperCollins, 2010.

Jung, Carl. *Memories, Dreams, and Reflections*. New York: Pantheon, 1963.

Harrington, Anne, *The Cure Within: A History of Mind-Body Medicine*. New York: W.W. Norton & Company, 2008.

Hogarth, Robin M. *Educating Intuition*. Chicago: University of Chicago Press, 2001.

Levy, Ze'ev. Edited by Greenberg, Yudit Kornberg. *From Spinoza to Lavinas: Hermeneutical, Ethical, and Political Issues in Modern and Contemporary Jewish Philosophy*. New York: Peter Lang Publishing, 2009.

Lipton, Bruce H., *The Biology of Belief: Unleashing the Power of Consciousness, Matter, & Miracles*. Carlsbad, CA: Hay House 2008.

Long, Jeffrey, and Perry, Paul, *Evidence of the Afterlife: The Science of Near-Death Experiences*. New York: HarperOne, 2010.

Mann, Thomas. *The Black Swan*. New York: Alfred A. Knopf, 1954.

Nuland, Sherwin B. *Maimonides*. New York: Schocken, 2008.

Siegel, Bernie S., MD, *Love, Medicine, & Miracles*. New York: Harper & Row, 1986.

Sloan, Richard P. *Blind Faith: The Unholy Alliance of Religion and Medicine*. New York: St. Martin's Griffin, 2008.

Sontag, Susan. *Illness as Metaphor*. New York: Farrar, Straus and Giroux, 1978.

Sternberg, Eliezer J. *Are You a Machine?: The Brain, the Mind, and What It Means to Be Human*. Amherst, NY: Humanity Books, 2007.

Thomas, Gordon. *Mysteries of the Human Body: Medical Miracles and Unexplained Phenomena of Human Biology*. London: Carlton Books, 2005.

Weil, Andrew. *Spontaneous Healing: How to Discover and Embrace Your Body's Natural Ability to Maintain and Heal Itself*. New York: Ballantine Books, 2000.

Williams, William Carlos. *The Doctor Stories*. New York: New Directions, 1984.

Index

Aaron (biblical), 184

Aberfan (Wales), landslide in, 68

Abramson Cancer Center, University of Pennsylvania School of Medicine, 106–107

adrenaline, mind-body effect and, 56

adult-onset diabetes, 30–31

allopathic medicine, 4

alpha interferon, 156

alternative medicine, 4, 167–172

"alter" personality, 34

Altman, Shem, 171–172

amygdala, 132

Anatomy of Hope, The (Groopman), 107

anger, mind-body effect and, 44–54

anoxia/anoxic encephalopathy
brain chemistry and, 25–26
chances of recovering from, 21

emotion and recovery, 25–27

examples of, 15–23

out-of-body experiences and, 19, 22–24

antibiotics, 88–94

anti-neoplastons, 163

antipsychotic medication, 80

antiviral treatment, 156

anxiety
depression in cancer patients, 107
mind-body effect and, 44–54
premonition and, 59–64
recognizing, 9–14
susceptibility/response to infection, 94

Ashkhabad (U.S.S.R.), earthquake in, 68

Augustine, St., 182–183

autologous vaccine, 108–109

Avastin, 108

Ayurveda, 13–14

bacteria, 92–94

Bausell, R. Barker, 170

Beaumont Hospital (Michigan), 178–182

Behavioral Oncology Program, Abramson Cancer Center, University of Pennsylvania School of Medicine, 106–107

Behm, David, 57

Bellevue (Siegel), 157

Bernheim, Hippolyte, 83

Berserkers, 56

beta blockers, 62, 63

Bierman, Dick, 69

birth control pills, 127–130

Black Swan, The (Mann), 121–122

Blackmore, Susan, 23

Blaine, David, 146–153

Blanke, Olaf, 23–24

Blind Faith (Sloan), 117–118

blood pressure, 60–64

blood sugar, 29–34, 37, 39–41, 84

Bourguignon, Erica, 82

brain
  premonition and, 69
  recovery from anoxia and, 23–24
  "state of mind" and, 40
  stress and, 132
  "superhuman strength" and, 54–57
  See also mind-body effect

breast cancer, 164–165, 167–169

breath, holding, 146, 148–153

Broad Institute, MIT/Harvard, 162

Brown University, 69–70

Burzynski, Stanislaw, 163

Calvinism, 100

cancer
  breast, 164–165, 167–169
  liver, 158–165
  lung, 61–64, 111–119, 175–176
  psychic healing for, 134–136
  will to live and, 106–109

Cancer Journal for Clinicians, 161

Cat's claw, 171

Cayce, Edgar, 134

Centers for Disease Control, 89

Central Park Jogger, The (Meili), 21

Charcot, Jean-Martin, 83

Chekhov, Anton, 157

chemoembolization, 159, 162

Child Study Center, New York University (NYU), 39

Christianity, 112. *See also individual Christian denominations*

cirrhosis, 156–165

Clarke, David C., 130–131

cleanliness, in hospitals, 92–93

Cleveland Clinic, 170

clindamycin, 90–91

Cohen, Mary Ann, 21

colon, infected, 96–106

coma
  brain chemistry and, 25–26
  chances of recovering from, 21
  emotion and recovery, 25–27
  examples of, 15–23
  out-of-body experiences and, 19, 22–24

Coma Recovery Association, 22

complementary and alternative
    medicine (CAM), 169–170. *See
    also* alternative medicine
conversion hysteria, 83
cortisol, 56. *See also* stress
Coyne, James, 106–107
creativity, 82
Cure Within, The (Harrington), 82
cycle of worry, 10

death, premonition of. *See*
    premonition
delusion, neurosis *vs.*, 12
Demato, Paulette, 22
"demonic possession," 80, 82–83
Depakote, 80, 81
depression, in cancer patients, 107.
    See also anxiety
diabetes, 29–34, 37, 39–41
diagnosing, patient as guide for, 73–85
*Diagnostic and Statistical Manual
    IV-TR* (DSM IV-TR), 37
disinfection, 92–94
dissociative identity disorder (DID)
    defined, 37–39
    diagnosing, 29–34
    inner pulse as fragmented, 34–37
    metabolic differences and, 37,
        39–41
doctors
    perspective of, 84–85
    stress-related illnesses and,
        130–132
    training of, 3–5
Dosa, David M., 69–70
Doyle, Sir Arthur Conan, 146

ductal carcinoma in situ, 169
Duffin, Jacalyn, 5

École Polytechnique Fédérale
    (Lausanne, Switzerland), 23–24
Educating Intuition (Hogarth), 4,
    84–85
Edwards, Harry, 133–134
Edwards, Lindsay, 57
Ehrson, Henrik, 23–24
Eikele (Haftorah reading), 116
electroconvulsive (shock) therapy, 74
emotion
    brain and, 25–27
    susceptibility/response to
        infection, 93–94
    See also fear
"energy," psychic healing and,
    137–141
epilepsy, 23
epinephrine, 63
estrogen, 125–130
excited delirium syndrome, 56–57
exorcism, 80, 82–83

faith, 111–119
False Alarm (Siegel), 10, 125
family stress
    inner pulse and, 9–14
    mind-body effect and, 46–54
    premonition and, 64–67
fear
    fight-or-flight reaction, 39–40
    overcoming, 92–94
    public reaction and, 87–92
    stress and, 132

Feit, Fred, 179–180, 192, 194
fertility issues, 128–130
fight-or-flight reaction, 39–40
Folkman, Judah, 159
follicle-stimulating hormone (FSH),
    125–126
foreboding. *See* premonition
fragmented inner pulse. *See*
    dissociative identity
    disorder (DID)
Frankl, Viktor, 13
free will, 100
Freud, Sigmund, 84
Fuina, Anthony, 135–136

Gahl, William, 85
Gassner, Father Johann Larryph, 83
gene-targeted therapy, 163
Geneva (Switzerland) Hospital, 23
George Williams College, 57
glucose
    mind-body effect, 56
    personality and, 37, 84
glycosylated hemoglobin (A1C), 32
goji berry, 171
Golgi tendons, 57
Gopinathan, Govindan, 13–14
Gottlieb, Scott, 93
Grave's disease, 78, 80
Grines, Cindy, 180–182
Groopman, Jerome, 107
Gruber, Michael, 107–108, 188–189

Haftorah, 116
hallucination, 67–68
Hammond, Kenneth, 3–4

hand washing, 92
Harrington, Anne, 26, 82
Harvard University, 107, 162
healing
    difficulty of, 12
    psychic healing, 133–141
    See also recovery
heart attack, 178–182, 192–195
heavy metals, 172
Henry IV (king of England), 83
hepatic encephalopathy, 157, 163
hepatitis, 156–165, 174–175
herbs, 171
Hogarth, Robin, 4, 84–85
Holden, Janice, 24
Holland, R. F., 183
Houdini, Harry, 145–146
Hume, David, 181, 183
humor, 11, 51
hyperthyroidism, 76, 80
hypnosis, 55, 83–84
hypothalmus-pituitary-adrenal
    (HPA) axis, 40
hysteria, hypnosis and, 83–84. *See
    also* mental health

Ikai, Michio, 57
Illness as Metaphor (Sontag), 164
impossibility, overcoming,
    146–153
infection, fear and, 89–94
infectious-disease precaution, 92
infertility issues, 128–130
inner pulse
    alternative medicine, 167–172
    awareness of, 9–14

defined, 1
faith and, 111–119 (*See also* religion; spirituality)
fear and, 87–94
as medical tool, 2–3
medical training, 3–5
mind-body effect, 43–57
miracles, 173–185
outliving prognosis, 155–165
personality and, 29–41
perspective, 73–85
premonition, 59–70
psychic healing, 133–141
recognizing, 187–195
recovery, 15–27
spiritual power of, 145–153
stress-related illnesses, 121–132
will to live, 95–109
Institute of Applied Biology, 161–162
Institute of Noetic Sciences, 69
insulin, 177
intensive care units (ICU), of hospitals, 19
intravenous gamma globulin (IVIG), 45
intuition
inner pulse as cognitive process, 4 (*see also* inner pulse)
negative intuition, 64 (*see also* premonition)

Jahuar, Sandeep, 26
Journal of Applied Physiology, 57
Journal of Clinical Oncology, 164–165

Journal of the American Medical Association, 161
Judaism
faith, 112–119
mitzvahs, 99, 182
soul, 100, 103–104
Jung, Carl, 22–23, 194–195
juvenile diabetes, 30–31

Kabbalah, 114
Karolinska Institute (Stockholm, Sweden), 23–24
Karten, Mitchell, 136
Kilham, Chris, 171
Kluft, Richard P., 38, 40–41
Korach (Torah), 184

lactulose, 157
Lamictal, 80
Lieberman, Rabbi Chanoch Hendel, 184–185
liver cancer, 158–165
liver failure, 156–165
Loewenstein, Richard J., 38
Long, Jeffrey P., 24
Love, Medicine, and Miracles (Siegel), 164
lung cancer, 61–64, 111–119, 175–176
lung capacity, holding breath and, 146, 148–153

Maimonides, Moses, 100, 118, 179
Making Rounds with Oscar (Dosa), 69–70

mania, hyperthyroidism and, 76, 80.
    See also mental health
Mann, Thomas, 121–122
Manning, Matthew, 134
Marescot, Michel, 83
marital stress. *See* family stress
Massachusetts Institute of
    Technology (MIT), 162
Medical Miracles (Duffin), 4–5
medical school, 3–5
Megibow, Alec, 181, 182
Meili, Trisha, 21
Memorial University of
    Newfoundland, 57
Memories, Dreams, and Reflections
    (Jung), 22–23
menopause, premature, 121–132
mental health
    anxiety, 9–14, 44–54, 59–64,
        94, 107
    dissociative identity disorder
        (DID), 29–41
    mind-body effect and, 44–54
    thyroid and, 73–82, 84
    See also mind-body effect
Mesmer, Franz Anton, 83
Messing, Wolf, 68
metals, 172
methicillin resistant staph aureus
    (MRSA), 88–94
mind-body effect
    examples, 44–54, 56
    excited delirium syndrome, 56–57
    non-linear nature of, 43–44
    thyroid and, 84
    trance and, 54–57

miracles
    faith and, 118–119
    kindness and, 182–185
    medicine and, 4–5
    religion and, 13
    reversing fortune and, 177–182
    sensitivity and, 173–177
mitzvahs, 99, 182
multiple personality disorder.
    See dissociative identity
    disorder (DID)
muscular dystrophy, 44–54

National Cancer Institute, 112
National Center of Complementary
    and Alternative Medicine
    (NIH), 169
National Institutes of Health, 169
    Undiagnosed Diseases
    Program, 85
near-death experiences (NDEs),
    19, 22–24
negative intuition, 64
neurosis, delusion *vs.*, 12
New England Journal of Medicine,
    69, 162
New York University (NYU),
    188–189
New York University (NYU) Child
    Study Center, 39
nitroglycerin, 193
noradrenaline, 56
norepinephrine, 63

Oprah, 149, 150
Orbito, Alex, 134–135

Orne, Martin, 55
Oscar (cat), 69–70
out-of-body experiences, 19, 22–24
ovaries, 126

Pachter, Leon, 104, 189–190
Padre Pio, Saint, 135–136
pain
    coma and, 17–18
    as indicator of health issues,
        2, 122
paranoia, worry and, 10–11
passion. *See* emotion
"performing muscles," 57
Perry, Bruce, 40
personality
    changes in, 29–37
    identity and, 37–39
    metabolic differences and, 37,
        39–41, 84 (*See also* dissociative
        identity disorder (DID))
perspective
    point of view and, 82–85
    recognizing problem and, 73–82
Posner, David, 148–149
"possession," 80, 82–83
premonition
    brain and, 69
    characteristics of, 67–68
    historical examples of, 68–70
    misplaced, 64–67
    as self-fulfilling prophecy, 59–64
progesterone, 127–130
psychic healing, 133–141
    authenticity of, 136–141
    examples of, 133–136

psychic surgeons, 134–135
psychosis, thyroid and, 73–82, 84
Pyramid of Asia Spiritual Healing
        Center (Cabanbanan,
        Manaoag), 135

Radin, Dean, 69
Ray, Andrew, 21–22
Ray, Emma, 21–22
recovery
    achieving balance, 13–14
    brain chemistry and, 25–26
    emotion and, 25–27
    examples of, 15–23
    nonlinear nature of, 43–44
    out-of-body experiences and, 19,
        22–24
reincarnation, 115
relaxation, 131, 167
religion
    Calvinism, 100
    Christianity, 112
    faith and, 111–119
    Judaism, 99, 100, 103–104,
        112–119, 182
    miracles and, 179, 180,
        182–185
    perspective and, 82
    recovery and, 13
    Roman Catholicism, 100
Revici, Emanuel, 160–162
Rhodiola rosea, 171
Robert Wood Johnson
        Foundation, 93
Roman Catholicism, 100
"running commentary" technique, 21

Sabon, Michael B., 24

Samson (biblical character), 56

Sandercock, Gavin, 56–57

Sarah (biblical), 121

Schneerson, Rabbi Menachem,
    65–66, 184–185

Science, 23

self-fulfilling prophecy, premonition
    and, 59–64

September 11, 2001 terrorist
    attacks, 56, 68–69

Shatkin, Jess P., 39

Shephard Pratt Health System
    (Baltimore, MD), 38

Showtime, 38

Siegel, Marc
    Bellevue, 157
    False Alarm, 10, 125

skin infection, 88–94

sleep, anxiety and, 10

Sloan, Richard, 117–118

SmithKline Beecham, 171

*Snake Oil Science: The Truth about
    Complementary and Alternative
    Medicine* (Bausell), 170

Sontag, Susan, 164

soul, 1, 100, 103–104

Spiegel, David, 107

"spiritualists," 146

spirituality
    faith and, 111–119
    openness to, 5
    perspective and, 82
    religion and, 13
    spiritual power of inner pulse,
        146–153

Stanford University, 107

Stargate (U.S. military), 69

Steinhaus, Arthur, 57

Stevenson, Ian, 68

stress
    cancer and, 165
    stress-related illness, 121–132

"superbugs," 87–94

"superhuman strength," 54–57

synchronicity, 194–195

Synthroid, 76–78, 81

Tanya (mystical text), 184

Temple University, 38

testosterone, 168

They Can't Find Anything Wrong
    (Clarke), 131

Thomas Aquinas, St., 183

thyroid, 73–82, 84

Titanic, 68

To Know and to Care, 185

Topalov, Andrei, 48–49

Torah, 184

trance, 54–57

Trauma Disorders Program,
    Shephard Pratt Health System
    (Baltimore, MD), 38

type 1/2 diabetes, 30–31

Undiagnosed Diseases Program
    (National Institutes of
    Health), 85

United States of Tara, The (Showtime
    series), 38

University of Amsterdam, 69

University of Maryland, 92

University of Pennsylvania School of
    Medicine, 106–107

Van Dyck, Richard, 38
Vonnegut, Kurt, 156
VU Medical Center
    (Amsterdam), 38

Ward Six (Chekhov), 157
will to live
    defying statistics and, 96–106
    quality of life and, 106–109
    religious views, 100, 103–104
Wittgenstein, Ludwig, 183
worry, 9–14. *See also* anxiety